the lesbian
Kama Sutra

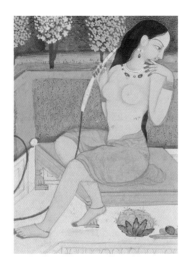

THOMAS DUNNE BOOKS
An imprint of St. Martin's Press

www.stmartins.com

Library of Congress Cataloging-in-
Publication Data available upon request

ISBN 0-312-33585-7
EAN 978-0312-33585-4

First published in the United Kingdom
by Carlton Books Limited
First U.S. edition: January 2005

10 9 8 7 6 5 4 3 2 1

Executive Editor: Lisa Dyer
Design: Axis Design Editions Ltd
Picture Manager: Steve Behan
Illustrator: Roger Payne
Production Controller: Janette Burgin

The author and publisher have made
every effort to ensure that all information
is correct and up to date at the time of
publication. Neither the author nor the
publisher can accept responsibility for
any accident, injury, or damage that
results from using the ideas, information,
and advice offered in this book.

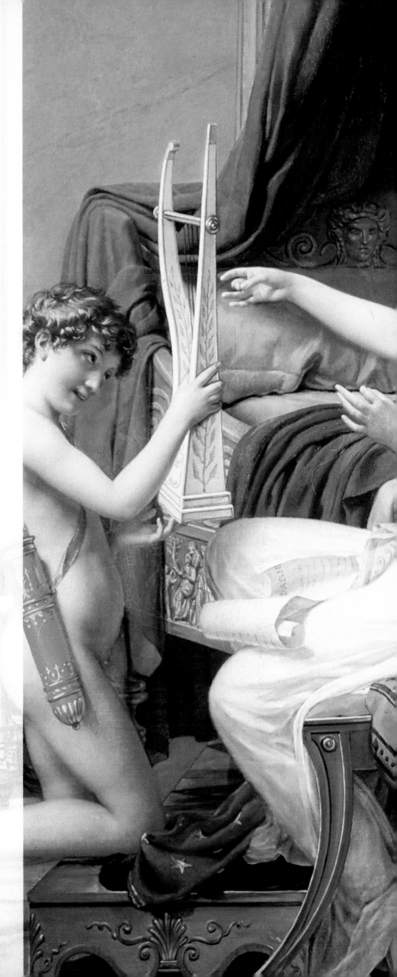

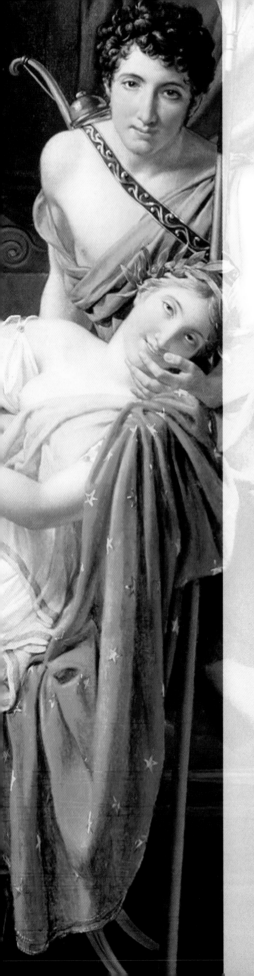

the lesbian
Kama Sutra

Thomas Dunne Books

St. Martin's Press ☙ New York

contents

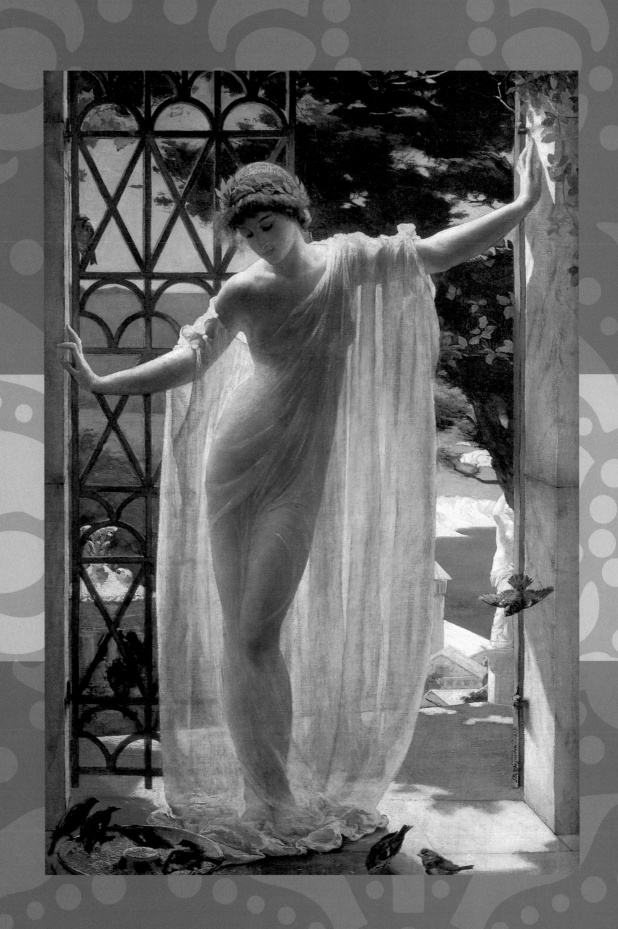

Chapter 1:
Introduction

history

Of the many manuals on love and sex written throughout the centuries, and across different cultures, the Kama Sutra is still regarded as the most famous and the most enduring of all.

While many people may not have read its pages from cover to cover, few will be unaware of the existence of the Kama Sutra, for it is renowned as an ancient, even mystical, guide that positively encourages experimentation with sexual positions and techniques. However, there is more to the Kama Sutra than the pursuit of acrobatic sex.

Compiled in the fourth century BC by the Hindu scholar Vatsyayana, the Kama Sutra was intended to be a manual for good and fulfilled living in a civilized society. As well as advocating exploration of sexual techniques and positions, Vatsyayana wanted to highlight a spiritual and religious dimension, too. Sex, he believed, was a fundamental human need, one that was not to be repressed, but rather enjoyed and practised thoroughly. However, he also noted that sexual energy is a powerful tool and while the Kama Sutra advocates uninhibited sexual enjoyment, the philosophy at its heart also advises that pleasures should be used for a higher or 'noble' purpose. According to Vatsyayana, we should use the Kama Sutra to understand the position of humanity, not only in this world but also as a fleeting moment in eternity.

OPPOSITE Although it has never been given the same prominence as heterosexual sex or men-only sex, physical intimacy between women has a rich history, as shown in this evocative eighteenth-century Pahari-style painting of girls bathing, from the Kanga School, Himachal Pradesh.

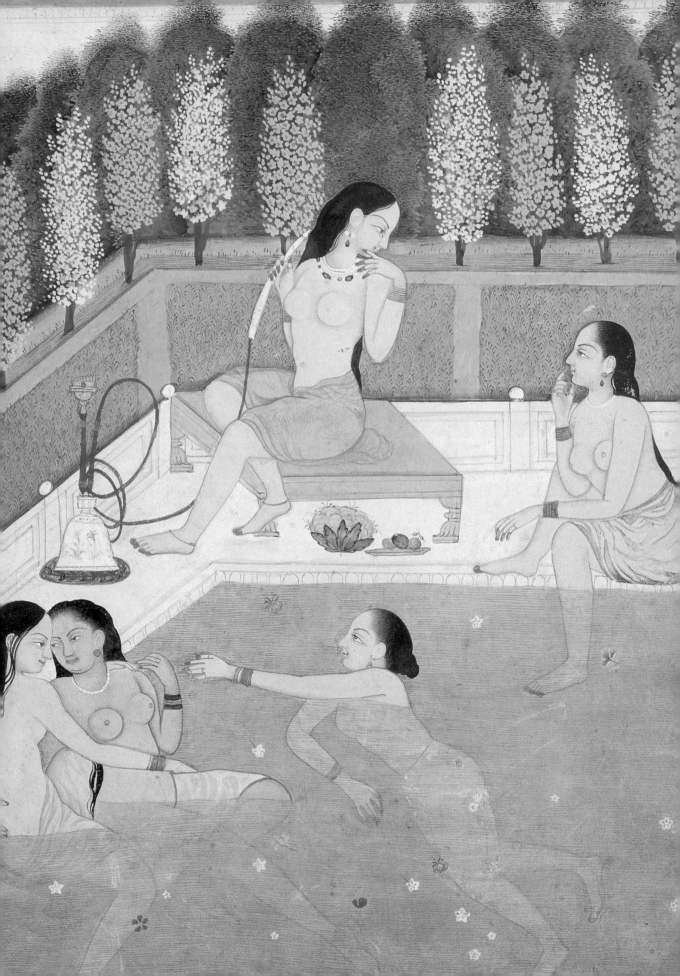

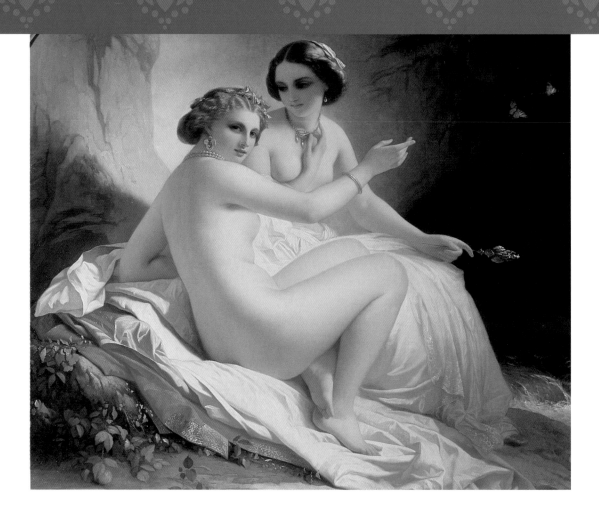

ABOVE Though not plentiful, strong portrayals of intimate relations between women have a firm place in art and literature, as seen here in 'The Bathers' (1830) by Louis Hersent. More often than not, such works were commissioned for men.

Originally written in Sanskrit, the title 'Kama Sutra' loosely translates into 'the rules of love'. The word '*kama*' means physical passion (and is the name of the lesser Hindu god who ruled over it), while '*sutra*' stands for aphorism, the expression of an idea in as few words as possible. And that is what the manual sets out to do – to provide rules for men and women on how to live their lives, how to relate to one another and how to create a civilized society.

In the Kama Sutra, male and female roles are clearly defined. Any woman reading the book cannot fail to see the emphasis is on the sexual gratification of the man (and some heterosexual women might argue how little things have changed in two millennia). The man's role is to be a perfect and experienced sexual partner, while the woman is to be dutiful to the man and to do everything in her power to please him. Although the Kama Sutra was written from a heterosexual viewpoint, sex and intimacy between couples of the same sex are given a small part in the manual.

A lesbian interpretation

India has always had an ambiguous relationship with gay sex. Sex between men was regarded as the domain of effeminates and eunuchs, yet it is clear from the Kama Sutra that it went on. Most gay sex, so the Kama Sutra informs us, is centred on oral gratification, invariably for money. Lesbian activity, too, is not ignored. Men enjoyed the dominant position in society and often had more than one wife, as well as mistresses and even concubines. The women of the harem were frequently left alone together for long periods of time, and Vatsyayana comments: 'Since the women of the harem are not allowed to other men and have one husband in common to all of them, they are physically dissatisfied and therefore give pleasure to each other'. He also tells of women being amorous and 'doing the acts of the mouth on the *yonis* [vaginas] of one another'. Vatsyayana continues to state that women should know the way of kissing the *yoni* because it is like kissing the mouth. There appears to be no judgement made on these acts of oral sex; rather Vatsyayana treats them as a fact of life.

Because the Kama Sutra is aimed at heterosexual couples and mention of lesbian sex is minimal, there is a temptation to ask what possible relevance it could have for us as lesbians, women who have sex with other women. In some ways, the manual is a

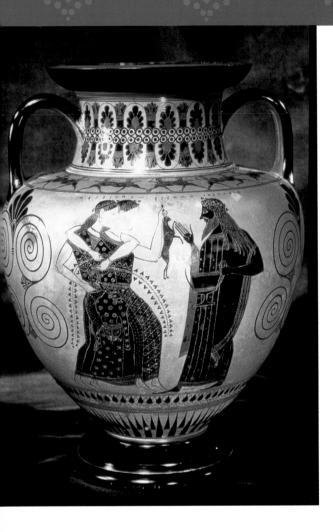

ABOVE Ancient societies were less judgmental than modern society when it came to expressions of same-sex love. Pottery artefacts depicting such images can be traced back over 2,500 years, predating the Kama Sutra itself. Here, an Attic amphora depicts a Dionysian scene with two women by an Amasis painter (c 540–530 BC).

reflection of the attitudes of society in general, from ancient times to the modern day; heterosexual relationships take precedence, and sex and intimacy between lesbian and gay couples is acknowledged fleetingly, and is not seen as being as important as straight sex. But there are a number of elements we can draw from the manual and use to our benefit. The Kama Sutra encourages honest and open exploration of human sexuality. It is almost 2,500 years old, yet it still has resonance for modern living. In fact, in these increasingly contradictory times, where opposition to homosexuality grows as our human rights become more enshrined in law, the manual has a message at its heart that is more important than ever: human sexual urges are natural and positive and, as such, individual sexual impulses are good and worthy.

Many of us have experienced the isolation that a difference in sexual orientation can create. We need reassurance that our impulses are as valid as those of heterosexuals, especially when there's a whole world out there just waiting to tell you that what you feel – and what you are – is wrong or immoral. The Kama Sutra harks back to an age when society wasn't perturbed about same-sex love and intimacy: women had sex with women and men had sex with men. No doubt, it has been like that since the creation of humanity.

In some cultures, same-sex love was practised more openly; in Indian culture, it has always been covert and with some legal penalty. The earliest surviving text on Indian law is the *Arthashatra*, a document from fourth century BC, which records fines given for gay and lesbian activities, though these are lower than the fines for certain heterosexual behaviour. Ironically, sex between people of the same sex was prohibited only if they were of different castes – the rigorous and ancient class system that divides India even today.

Ancient societies

In some ways, ancient society was more enlightened about sexual differences than we are in modern times. In the past, some societies celebrated sex and sexuality as a force of strength and fertility. Like India and China, and Japan to a lesser degree, the Celtic countries and Roman cultures had a tradition of art and literature depicting sex, lesbian and gay sex included.

When it came to same-sex desire, probably one of the most tolerant countries was ancient Greece, where no laws existed to condemn lesbian love and homosexual desire was an unremarkable, everyday emotion. Two hundred years before the Kama Sutra was written, in the sixth century BC, the most famous lesbian of them all, the poet Sappho, ran an all-female educational and

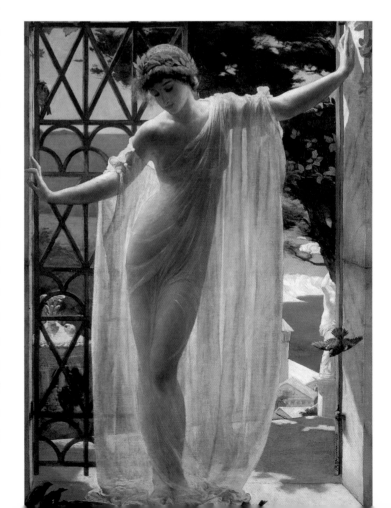

BELOW 'Lesbia' by John Reinhard Weguelin (1849–1927), an image of Grecian beauty inspired by the female cult of Lesbos.

social community on the Greek island of Lesbos. Hers was just one of many *thiasos*, a type of finishing school, where older women trained teenage girls in art, music, dance and beauty, in supposed preparation for marriage. Here, they worshipped the goddess Artemis, the Roman Diana, who was often depicted in erotic closeness with her female followers. Rituals honouring Artemis would be conducted, and the women would anoint one another and cover each other in floral garlands. Although Sappho herself was married, her poetry pays homage to her love objects, among them some of her pupils. It was the passion of her poetry, to and about women, that gave rise to the term 'lesbian', deriving from Sappho's homeland of Lesbos. Academics argue that the term didn't take on its current sexual connotations until around 900 years later, and the term 'Sapphist' has been used throughout recent centuries to mean any woman who preferred the company of other women or spent intimate time with them.

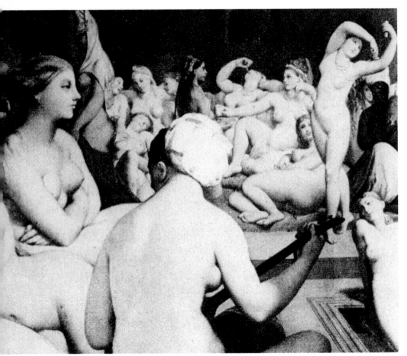

ABOVE The sensuous masterpiece 'The Turkish Bath' by Jean-Auguste-Dominique Ingres (1780–1867) depicts a group of women enjoying music, dance and each other's company. In many cultures harem women were left alone together for long periods and it was then that they turned to each other for comfort and sexual pleasure.

Such honesty or even neutrality to sexual difference is now long gone. Prescriptions and prejudices, often strengthened by the fundamentalist views of some modern-day religions, now replace the sexually and emotionally open and honest societies of an apparently golden era, which allowed Sappho her schools and enabled the Kama Sutra to be written. In the time since the Kama Sutra was compiled, society has changed: civilizations have come and gone, religions flourished and died. Some of Vatsyayana's teachings have stood the test of time in relation to modern culture, others have not. As women in the Western world, we can no longer identify with the often-restrictive rules that govern the lives and sexuality of women, while attitudes towards lesbianism and homosexuality are now changing quickly, year by year.

In 1883, when the Kama Sutra was translated by Sir Richard F Burton and F F Arbuthnot, the two men decided that only a few copies should be printed as the book might cause controversy in Victorian England. It was not until the 1960s – another 80 years on – that society at large was allowed to see the book when it finally went on general release. Today we cannot pretend that centuries of learning and scientific progress have not happened and that the quality of our lives and health has not improved. However, the core philosophies of this ancient text – peace, love, tolerance and open expression – are ones we should, and can, embrace. They are still important virtues which, if practised, will allow us to find the honesty to deal with our own needs, wants and sexual desires, free from shame or embarrassment.

Sappho, if you will not get up and let us look at you,
I shall never love you again.
Get up, unleash your suppleness, lift off your Chian nightdress.
The gods bless you.
May you sleep then,
On some tender girl friend's breast.

SAPPHO, QUOTING HER STUDENT ATTHIS

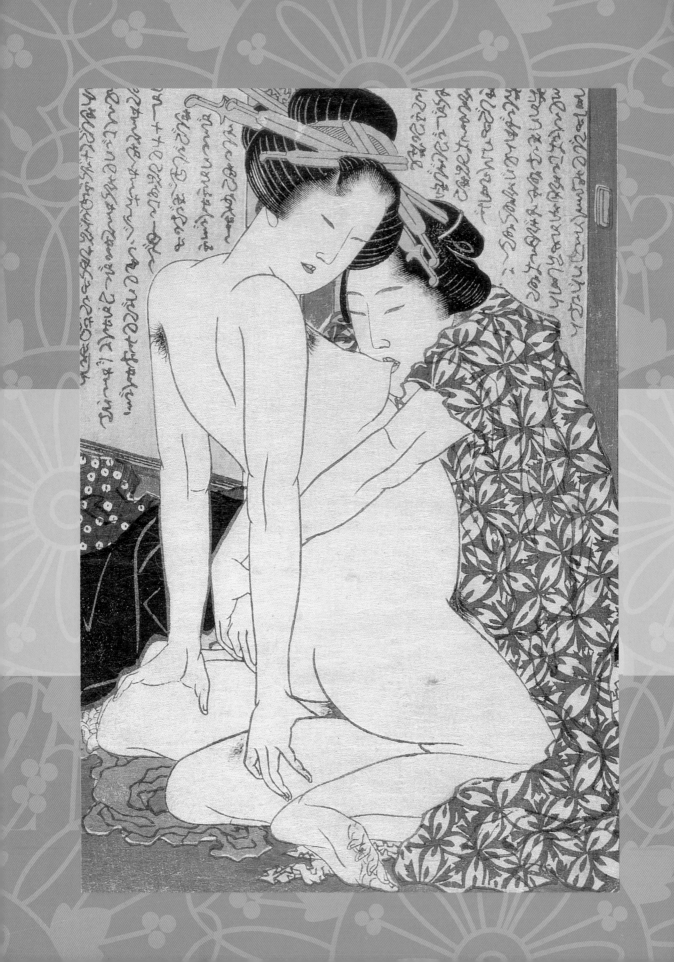

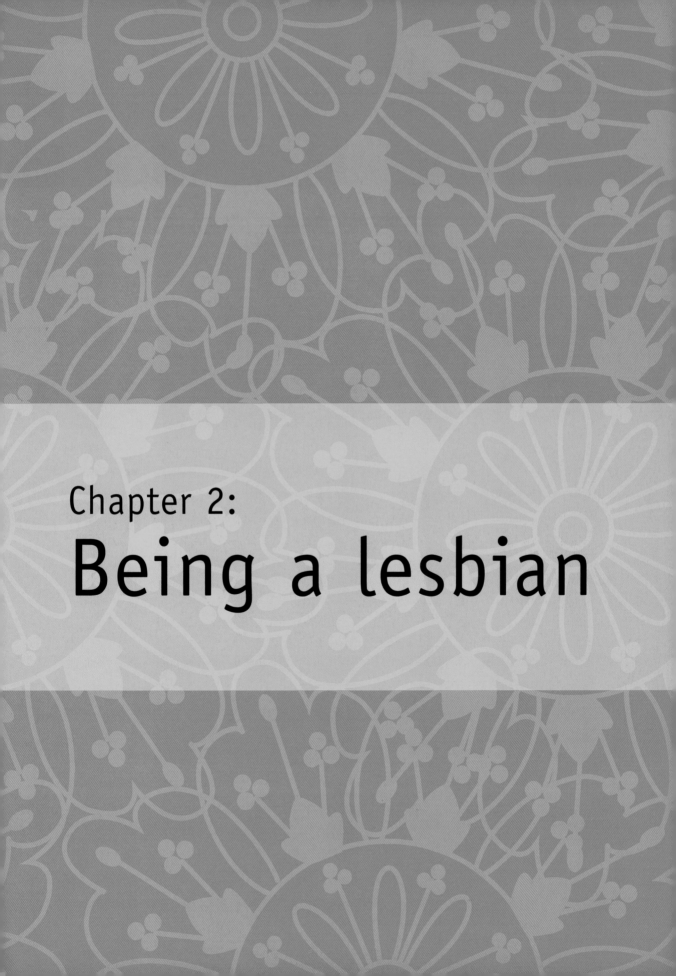

Chapter 2:
Being a lesbian

the lesbian image

Sexuality is the force that drives the natural world and it's an important factor in the character of all humans. Lesbianism is the sexual and emotional intimacy between women and, like gay relationships, it is universal.

Lesbianism has been practised since ancient times and throughout the world. Evidence of it is reflected in images of same-sex love, spanning thousands of years across a variety of cultures.

Everyone wants to see visual representation of their own lives, and none more so than lesbians and gay men, especially when they are made to feel or believe by society that what they are is wrong and, worse, that they never existed.

How many of us can remember being a teenager, knowing we were sexually attracted to other women, but not knowing what to do with that emotion? Remember how confused you felt back then and how vulnerable, too? Then, there was frustration because your friends and peers weren't feeling this way; they were dating boys, and you didn't dare tell them about the girl you fancied because they might reject you or even turn against you because of it. From my own experience, and I can't imagine I am alone, it was then that I desperately sought images – a story in a magazine, a book or even a TV programme – which might, just briefly, reflect what I was

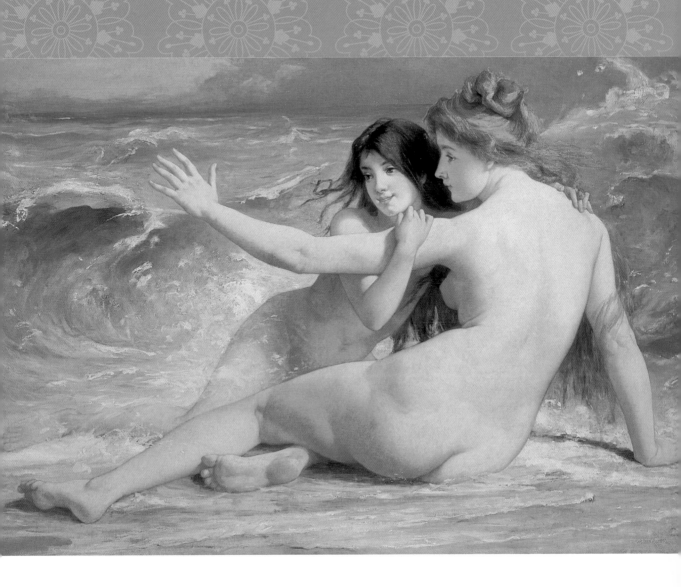

feeling, and it would prove that there were other women with these feelings. It was important to know that I wasn't alone with a very powerful and raw emotion, even though there was no one to talk to. This is why images of intimacy between women are important to us. They illustrate centuries of sex, love and relations between women; they show us we have always existed. Visibility is an important aspect in the validation of the lesbian identity.

Over the past two decades, lesbians in the Western world have become more visible than we have been since, perhaps, ancient Greece, when Sappho's schools for women and lesbian art existed. At that time, images of emotional intimacy between women were

ABOVE 'Les Baigneuses' by Paul Albert Laurens (1870–1934). Although lesbian love has been illustrated in previous centuries, over the past two decades we, as lesbians, have been responsible for creating our own images, which empowers us and strengthens our identity.

created by women themselves through art and poetry. Such female bonding was seen as a fact of life. Now that lesbianism as a valid social constituent has finally emerged from its own dark ages, we create our own images – in art, film, literature, business, the media, entertainment, and in all aspects of life – which gives us more control over our identity and our representation.

The last few decades have seen the social mores that kept us static and hidden shift and shatter, and we enjoy a greatly improved level of self-worth and image. Traditionally, literature has been littered with negative images of lesbians. And while there have been a few rare works of fiction in which lesbians were represented in a positive way – notably Patricia Highsmith's revolutionary 1950s novel, *Carol* (also released under the title *The Price of Salt*) – most books before the 1970s were written with an eye to the censors, invariably ending with the female protagonists being married, killed off or sectioned to an asylum.

With the burgeoning of lesbian fiction, the work of lesbian authors has become widely accessible. Indeed, Rita Mae Brown's *Ruby Fruit Jungle* and Jeanette Winterson's *Oranges Are Not the Only Fruit* are now considered literary classics, while Sarah Waters' explicitly sexual *Tipping the Velvet* (2002) was made into a BBC television drama in the UK and shown worldwide. Such films as *Desert Hearts* (1986), *Go Fish* (1994) and *The Incredibly True Adventures of Two Girls in Love* (1995), to name but a few, have significantly shaped lesbian identity and its image in the world. Commercial lesbian magazines are easily available, such as *Curve* and *Girlfriend* in the USA, *Diva* in the UK and *Lesbians on the Loose* in Australia, thus allowing us increased awareness of ourselves and the diversity in our identities.

Aimed at the gratification of straight men, images of lesbian sex have long been a mainstay of pornography. However, over the last ten years or so, lesbians have begun to take control of their own sexual image, and it is now possible to buy erotic magazines, books and films to whet every female appetite – from softcore porn to hardcore S&M acts. Accurate and realistic depictions of lesbian life, love and sex are now conveyed in books and magazines and on television and film, which show the world that lesbians can be any 'type' of woman. These images allow us to escape from the restrictive stereotypes that heterosexual men have given, and in some situations forced upon, us.

The hidden history

One of the most famous poets of her era, as well as a fine artist, Sappho naturally emphasized art and poetry at her all-female communities in ancient Greece, and her relationships with other women were reflected in those works. Her attraction to the same sex, and her love of her pupils, was not seen as unusual and elicited no disapproval; it even succeeded in drawing women travellers from other parts of Europe to pay homage. In his book, *Pictures and Passions: A History of Homosexuality in the Visual Arts*,

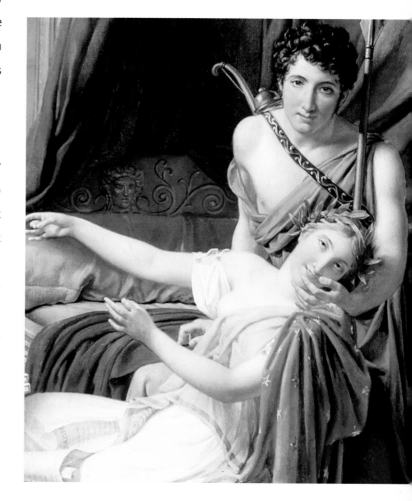

BELOW 'Sappho and Phaon' by Jacques-Louis David, *c* 1809. Sappho was the most famous poet of her era and ran all-female schools. Her adoration of, and relationships with, other women was not seen as unusual, and reflected the more tolerant attitudes of ancient Greece.

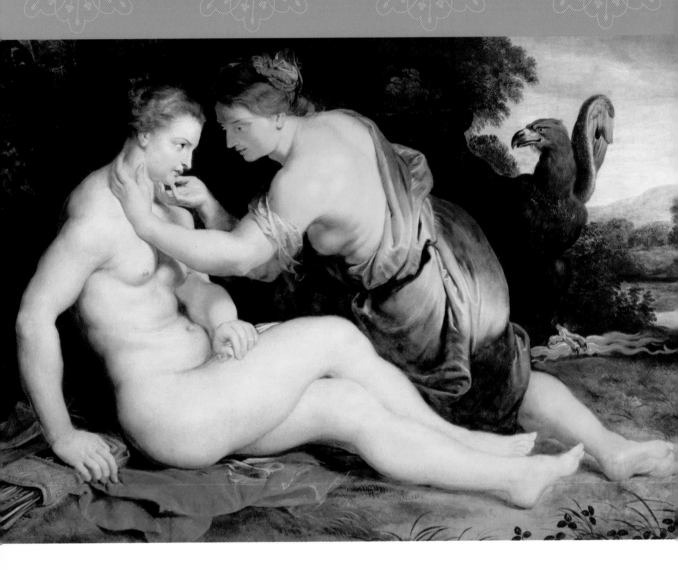

ABOVE 'Jupiter and Callisto', c 1613, by Peter Paul Rubens (1577–1640). In Roman mythology, one of Diana's companions, Callisto, lost her virginity to Jupiter, who was disguised as Diana. In her rage, Diana turned Callisto into a bear and placed her in the sky as the constellation Ursa Major, the Great Bear.

James M Saslow indicates that Sappho became a cultural icon. In fact, several statues, paintings and the coins of her native city of Mytilene paid tribute to her image. Saslow also indicates that, after her death in around 540 BC, Sappho had no artistic or literary successors and her influence gradually disappeared so that by the sixth century, Greek women largely became confined to their domestic roles. After Sappho virtually all literature was produced by men and, as lesbian sex and relations didn't involve them, Greek writing no longer touched upon these subjects. However, legends of all-female societies and tribes remained. One lasting fable was the Amazons, a mythical and fearless tribe of women warriors around the time of 400–440 BC, who renounced men in order to live together in a sexually charged atmosphere. Of large, muscular proportion, these female warriors were said to live in Asia Minor (modern Turkey), where they worshipped the goddess Artemis (the Roman Diana), and the historian Herodotus gives an account of battles between Greek soldiers and an army of such women at the Black Sea. So enamoured were some men by the supposed strength and success in battle of the Amazonian women that the tribe was depicted in public sculptures. Though admired, painted and sculpted, the Amazons were also viewed as threatening, so were never portrayed as being entirely victorious.

For many centuries, Artemis/Diana, the goddess of the moon, has been associated with and worshipped by women because of her links with fertility and childbirth. She is frequently portrayed surrounded by her female devotees. Images of the goddess as Diana, with her attendant, Callisto, can be found in Roman art. Many illustrations of Diana and Actaeon, the male hunter who met a bloody end after he stumbled upon Diana frolicking with her attendants, have appeared on floor mosaics, some dating back to the third and fourth centuries. Images of Diana and her devotees became quite commonplace in the sixteenth century; they were an illicit way of portraying titillating images of semi-clad women, often frolicking together, without offending propriety or the censors.

While sex between women went on throughout time, probably most often in the domestic environment, there is very little to see and read about female lovemaking from the time of Sappho until the sixteenth century. The proof that men did not treat sex, relations or physical intimacy between women seriously comes in Saslow's account of the rediscovery of Sappho's poetry by French scholars in the sixteenth century. Despite it being clear that the subjects of Sappho's affection in the poems were women, the academics refused to acknowledge this and instead reinterpreted the subjects as men for the publication of the work. And those men who were interested in sex between women were as fascinated then as straight men have been throughout history – treating us as fantasy fodder for their own gratification.

Many of the images that we would now describe as lesbian-orientated were intended, if not as a blatant pornography, then as

BELOW 'The Tepidarium', *c* 1853, by Theodore Chasseriaus (1819–56). Over the last five centuries many images of women together were not painted for women themselves, but rather for the gratification of men. The artworks invariably show many naked women together at some private activity, often touching or embracing.

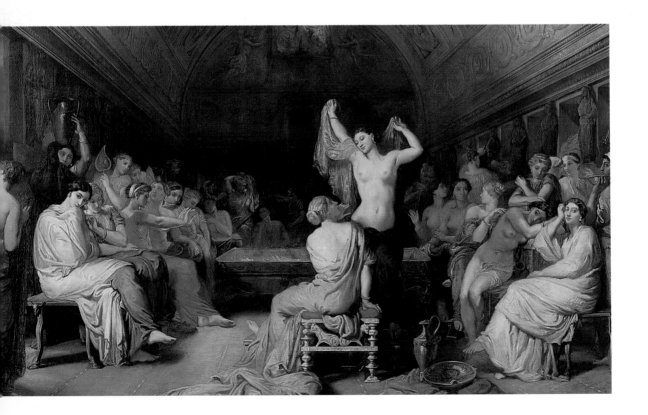

thrilling images. They were created *by* men *for* men and would sometimes be commissioned pieces of work. These works of art invariably show women together at some private activity, making the man an innocent (supposedly unintentional) voyeur of a clandestine female scene. A particularly favourite setting was the bathhouses, which involved many naked women, often embracing, sexually cavorting and fondling each other. Jean Mignon's 'Women Bathing' (1540) takes the voyeur into a sensuous world, where the female bathers are touching. In one coupling, a woman is clearly seen fondling the crotch of the other. In Titian's 'Diana and Actaeon' (1559), the nymphs and Diana bathe nude together. Women hidden away together, and the potential sexual play they might get up to – or rather,

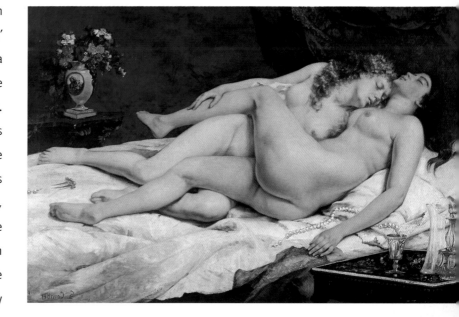

ABOVE 'The Sleep', c 1866, by Gustave Courbet (1819–77). Many of the titillating images of women caught together in an intimate moment or involved in risqué behaviour have been painted with the intention of making the man who stumbles upon the scene an innocent and unintentional voyeur.

what men would *fantasize* they might get up to – remained a theme in art well into the nineteenth century, other notable works on the subject being Jean-Auguste-Dominique Ingres' 'The Turkish Bathhouse' (1859–62). Men would not have seen inside these bathhouses, so painted scenes came from the imagination.

A great deal of the sexual imagery that exists of women together comes as a direct result of extensive movement across the world in the mid-sixteenth century. This was the time when

European travellers came into contact with female and male homosexuality and sexual expression across the continents. Often living in puritanical times back home – witch hunts across the Continent and the Inquisition in Spain, to name but two consequences, Europeans enforced their own sexual morality on the strange and new countries they visited. An eternity of sexual tolerance and practice disappeared overnight as countries were forced to abandon their natural outlook on same-sex intimacy and bring in laws with severe penalties for those found engaging in it.

In her book, *The Renaissance of Lesbianism in Early Modern England*, Valerie Traub tells of the sometimes-disturbing accounts of travellers, dignitaries and conquerors. The supposedly shocking, depraved sexual acts that were rumoured or relayed to these visitors were, however, often anecdotal and had sometimes been passed on through several people before being put in print. Nicholas de Nicholay, in his account of travels in Turkey, tells how the women of the bathhouses washed each other and become so 'fervently in love' that one woman might 'handle and grope another everywhere at their pleasure'. Thomas Glover, secretary to the English ambassador of Turkey, reported on the 'unnatural and filthy lusts' that were committed daily by women with women. There are accounts, too, of African women possessed by demons, having sex together, from French surgeon Ambroise Paré. (As if to reinforce the idea of African women's supposed lechery, Titian's painting 'Diana and Actaeon', shows Diana being towelled intimately by an

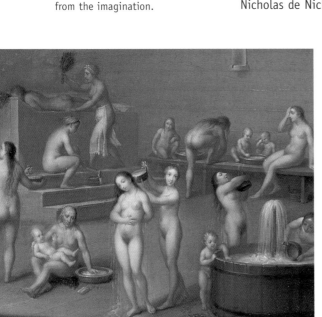

BELOW 'Russian Bath', *c* 1825, by Letunov (1814–41). Bathhouse settings were favoured by artists wanting to depict images of women naked and frolicking together. Men would not have been allowed inside, so everything shown came from the imagination.

African attendant.) But the most 'frightening' women of all were the 'tribade': monstrous figures who abused their own bodies and those of other women, penetrating them with their enlarged clitorises or with dildos. Mythical figures from classical literature, the tribade were introduced into Western society as a 'real' concept in the mid-sixteenth century (the time, Traub claims, when the medical profession rediscovered the importance of the clitoris in women's erotic pleasure). The term, a French expression derived from '*tribas*', the Greek for 'to rub', later came to refer to sexual acts between women. In English, those engaging in such acts were known as 'rubsters'. Though the word thankfully fell out of use when it came to describing lesbians, 'tribadism' remains – it's the practice of a woman rubbing her vagina against the vagina of another.

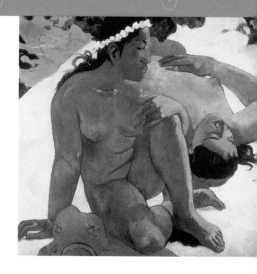

ABOVE 'Are You Jealous?' ('Aha oe feii?'), *c* 1892, by Paul Gauguin (1848–1903). Many images of intimacy between women come as a result of global travel.

The increase in travel, which continued into the seventeenth century and beyond, played an important role in the proliferation of lesbian images. It is because of the findings of the Renaissance travellers that we know of the rich imagery of lesbian sex and sexuality in art, artefacts and literature. James M Saslow refers to silk screens of lesbian sex and all-female threesomes from China, as well as Koka Pandita's *Koka Shastra*, another Indian sex manual of positions, dating from the twelfth century (though illustrated and translated in the seventeenth century for India's Islamic conquerors, the Moguls). In this publication, among all the pages of finely illustrated straight-sex acts, a particularly graphic image of lesbian sex is shown, in which one woman penetrates the open vagina of her lover with a dildo.

And in Nepal, where Hindu and Buddhist cultures overlap, Saslow tells of a carving discovered in the roof struts of a nineteenth-century shrine to the Hindu God, Shiva, standing in the

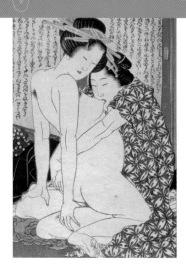

ABOVE A Chinese 'Shunga' (erotic) print of lesbian lovers, from 'Manpoku Wago-Jin', a colour woodblock, *c* 1821, by Katsushika Hokusai (1760–1849). Global travel and exploration brought Oriental and Asian imagery of lesbian sex and sexuality in art, literature and artefacts to the West.

capital Kathmandu, which shows one woman stimulating the vagina of her smiling female companion. During the British rule of Nepal (1816–1947), Queen Victoria's government closed down the erotic temples and some of the images were eventually defaced as obscene. In Victorian Britain, strict laws were enforced against male homosexuality, making it illegal and an imprisonable offence. Ironically, the same laws were never enforced against lesbian activity because the Queen could not bring herself to believe that women would do such things to one another. These views banished lesbian women into obscurity, and only served to further increase the ignorance surrounding same-sex love. This attitude wasn't, and still isn't, restricted to British society. Like generations of lesbian women before us, today's women who have sex with other women encounter intolerance wherever they live.

Dispelling the myths

Opinions held by society at large concerning lesbians and sex between women can, at best, be demoralizing and, at worse, outright offensive. Often people have an idea based on stereotyping about what it means to be lesbian or to be a gay man, which stems from a lack of informed knowledge. Gay men are often perceived to be effeminate and to hate women, and are regarded as weaker and more sensitive than their straight male counterparts. This is because the media, literature and the press have portrayed gay men in this way in a bid to make homosexuality non-threatening and non-masculine and, therefore, completely alien. Lesbians suffer from stereotyping and, similarly, find themselves misrepresented and misunderstood. There are frequent myths about lesbians and women who sleep with other women, which we have all, no doubt, encountered at some time. Here are a few of them.

Lesbians don't like men

Because we share physical and emotional intimacy, and build relationships with other women, it doesn't mean we don't like men – we simply choose not to have sex with them. Many women, however, will have had sexual relationships with men in the past, and they may even have been married or had children before taking a personal decision to come out about their sexuality and live openly as a lesbian. We are all different, and some women choose not to have too much contact with men – straight or gay – while others enjoy close and fulfilling friendships.

These days many gay women also choose to co-parent with male friends. It is likely that the idea we don't like men stems from men themselves. Lesbianism is guaranteed to make any straight man feel very insecure, unless it involves him – which it almost never does.

Lesbians want to be men

Just because lesbians sleep with women, this in no way means we want to be men. It's a long-held belief about lesbians, and one that plays itself out time and time again in media stereotypes: we are portrayed as aggressive, shaven-headed and extremely masculine – an opposite to the way gay men are pictured. As long as we're shown in this negative way, we're easier to discount and dismiss, and so we are not thought of as real women. I would be hard-pressed to think of any lesbians I've known or met in 15 years who actually want to be men. Again, this theory seems to originate from a male insecurity about lesbians and the utter incomprehension as to why a woman would want to sleep with another woman instead of a man.

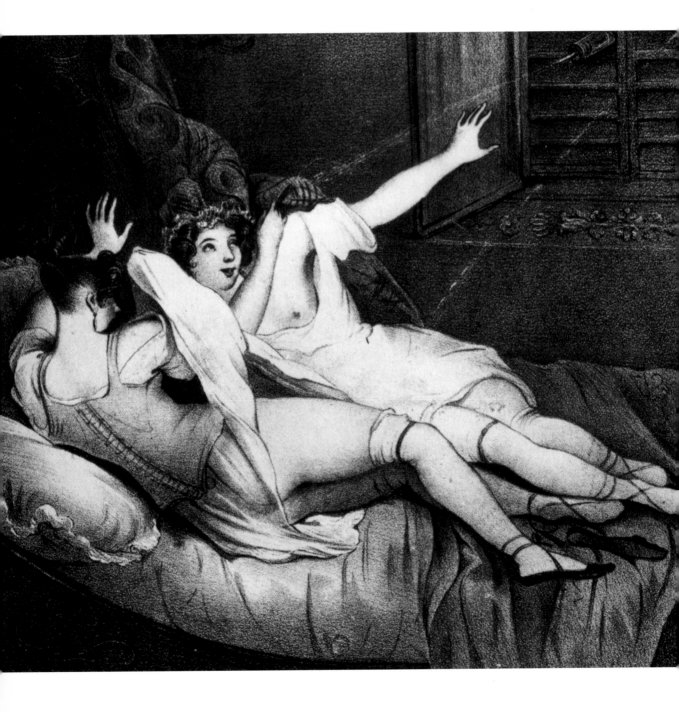

Lesbians don't like sex

For me, the most infuriating question I can ever be asked as a lesbian is probably the most clichéd. Exactly what do lesbians do in bed? Not only does the question show that the person asking it – whether a man or woman – has absolutely no imagination, but also that they have no idea of female anatomy and how a women responds to sexual stimulation. Because no one in that bed has a penis, it's assumed that we can't have sex. How many of us have met people who tell us they think all lesbians must do in bed is hug and that we are frigid? Wrong, wrong, wrong. Lesbians have hot, horny and extremely fulfilling sex in a myriad of different ways, which we'll see in detail in later chapters.

Lesbians don't have 'proper' sex

'Proper' or 'real' sex is thought to involve a man, and because lesbian sex doesn't, it is assumed not to be good or satisfying. Which leads to the next inaccuracy: that we all use dildos as artificial penises in a bid to try and reconstruct the heterosexual sex act. There's no one definitive way to have sex and lesbians, in my experience, are very inventive lovers; women's bodies and sexual responses offer a whole host of erotic possibilities. Yes, some women do use dildos, while others do not; some use sex toys, others penetrate their lovers, and some do not. There are lesbians who like anal sex and others who can't bear the thought of it. Some women enjoy rough sex, while others favour a tender and gentler sexual experience. It's all part of a widely diverse sexual identity.

OPPOSITE 'Two Lesbians in Bed', a lithograph from the early 1800s. Lesbians often suffer prejudice and stereotyping from society. Having confidence in yourself and your sexuality will help you to develop your own way of coping with any prejudice against you.

Something must have happened to make us like this

There are several arguments here. First, something bad happened to us and now we don't like men. This can be the reason why some women turn to their own sex. Something may have happened in their past history that has tried their trust in men, and now they feel safer with women. Others argue that they've been let down by men and so have turned to women instead. The other great continuing debate is the nature/nurture argument – whether we are born gay or whether we're gay because we choose to be so. Although I know some women care about what determines our sexual orientation, I personally don't: I just am a lesbian. To me, the most important factor is happiness and if being with another woman and having sex with her makes you happy, just do it. Life is very short. You get one chance, and at whatever time of your life you make the decision that this is what you want, grab it.

Lesbians are after every woman they meet

Feeling the discomfort of straight women is something most of us have experienced at one time or another. A sudden change in someone's attitude when they realize you're a lesbian is, no doubt, something with which we can all identify. Many straight people seem to think that lesbians and gay men are sexually insatiable and that we can't wait to get our hands on them. Invariably, they must also think us rather desperate, as even the least-attractive people can imagine you have a burning desire to have sex with them if you are gay. Yes, there are straight women we fancy – we see them in everyday life, in magazines and on television – but we are not necessarily going to act on our desires. In the same way, straight women don't make moves on every man they meet. Lesbians differ considerably from gay men in their sexual attitudes. Whereas some gay men think very little about picking up or having sex with a straight man (some actively look for it), lesbians are predominantly more inclined to look for women they know are sexually interested in other women. It's less complicated and more of a turn-on.

BELOW Lesbian venues, bars and clubs, as well as support networks and social groups, enable women to make contact with each other, something that can seem difficult to do when you're coming out.

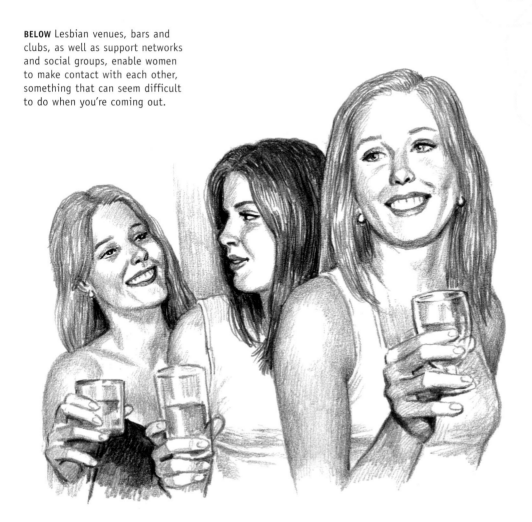

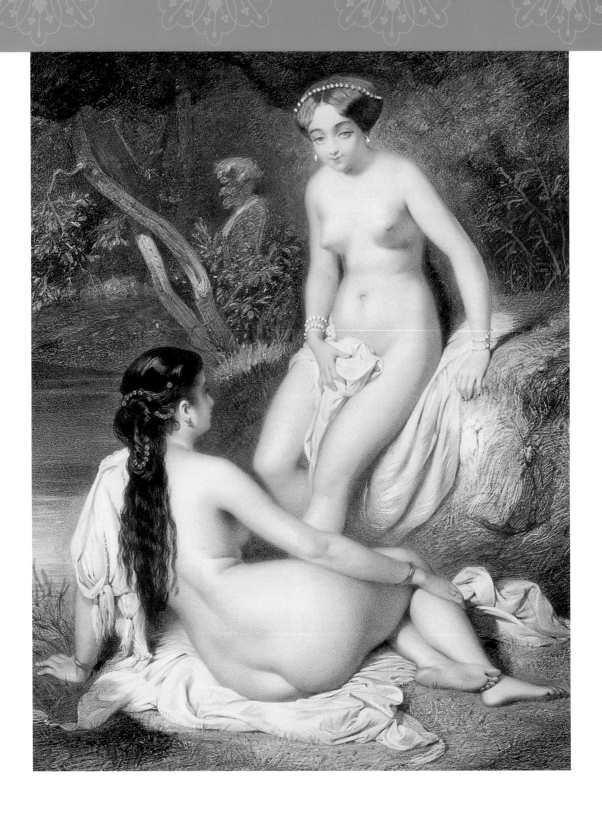

Raising self-esteem

While it's important to dispel these common myths, it's also vital not to allow them to affect the image we have of ourselves. Yes, we hear all kinds of ignorant things said about lesbians, and it takes each of us time and the benefit of experience to work through them all. But we *can* and eventually *do* work through them, and that's because it's all part of the growing-up process we undergo. It's a time of self-discovery which starts when we take the first few unsure steps out of that emotional and sexual closet – at whatever age that may be – and hopefully end up happy and fulfilled with the lifestyle and sexual choices we've made.

To conquer any negative feelings we may have about our sexuality, we must first raise our self-esteem levels. Whatever our sexual preferences, self-esteem is a crucial tool in the development of happy and well-rounded individuals, lovers and partners. As we know, some people can try to make us feel bad about being a lesbian and being 'different'. Religious groups may tell us we're evil, society might say we don't deserve the same rights as straight people, and our parents may even tell us how disappointed they are in us. But if we examine the ways in which we've been made to feel bad about our sexuality, we can challenge any doubts we have. One way to achieve this is to be certain that what we feel for other women is legitimate and valuable, emotionally and sexually; being honest and open with ourselves, as the Kama Sutra counsels. We must look at our lesbianism in a new and positive light, and some guidelines are featured overleaf.

OPPOSITE 'Conversation' or 'Two Bosom Friends' by Charles Bargue (1826–83). Seeing positive representations of lesbian women helps to raise self-esteem. It also allows women coming to terms with their sexuality to see how diverse we are as lesbians and how rich our history is.

OPPOSITE 'Girlfriends', 1913, by Egon Schiele. A happy and healthy relationship can bring each woman comfort and a sense of wellbeing.

● Educate yourself about your sexuality. Read from the extensive amount of literature available in a bid to understand the history, politics, struggles and triumphs of the lesbian world. Choose a few of the many resources that look at lesbian sexuality in a positive way (see also page 144).

● Seek out positive role models – women who live happy and fulfilled lesbian lifestyles. This does not necessarily mean women who are in couples, but anyone who embraces her identity and sexual desires openly and honestly. There are many sportswomen, artists, writers, filmmakers and other professionals in the public eye who might inspire you, but it could equally be someone you know.

● Learn to respect others and search out relationships where you are equal to the person you are with. This will lessen any feelings of self-doubt or worthlessness. Learning to be more assertive is also an important factor. The art of love is also that of communication. Assertiveness enables us to make our own feelings clear to a lover or partner and should provide the means for more effective and honest exchanges between people.

● Try positive reinforcement. You can improve the way you think about yourself and your desires by creating small, uplifting messages about your sexuality and repeating them every day. For example: 'My sexuality is a positive thing and I am not ashamed of who I am', or 'I will value and explore being a lesbian'. Write them down and place these messages of affirmation on a mirror so that you'll see them regularly – and repeat them every morning before you go out to face the world.

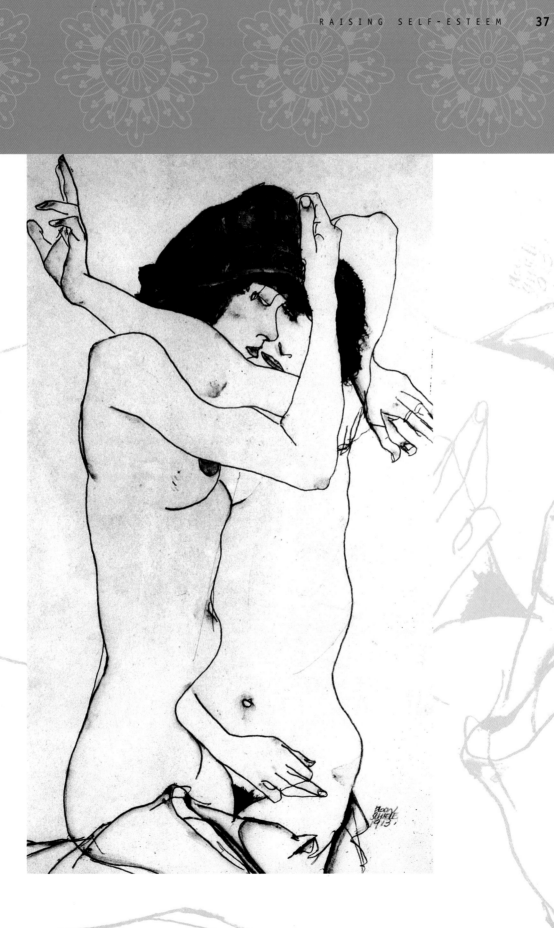

Lesbian sex and sexuality

Healthy self-esteem can improve your sex life, just as a good sex life can improve your self-esteem – the two are mutually bound together. While the actual sex you have with other women is a vastly important part of being a lesbian, it is not, however, the entirety of your sexuality. There is a difference between sex and sexuality.

Sex is a force that drives the world; the urge to come together with another person in pleasure being one of the strongest emotions. It's where you lay ourselves bare to someone else. It's when you can be at your most powerful, your most exciting and your most reckless, but you can also find yourself at your most vulnerable. Having sex is not just a means to an end – of only having an orgasm. Every woman needs to feel desired and wanted, and often invests a whole set of emotions in the lead-up, during and after the act of sex.

While it's accepted that men, on the whole, have a higher sex drive than women, women's sexual appetites have long been underestimated. It's true that each of us has very different needs and responses, and these can vary at particular times in our lives. Some women may have incredibly high sex drives, others moderate and some may experience a very low level of desire. None of these states is the right or wrong way to be; we are individuals and in sex, like everything else, we have different tastes.

How you approach finding sex also varies from woman to woman. Some women feel happy to go to a bar and pick up a woman for a one-night stand; others need to get to know their potential lover before they head for the bedroom. Again, there is no right and wrong in the way we find our sexual partners. However, it isn't always possible to get sex when you want it. For gay men, sex is easy to find. By going 'cottaging' (seeking sex in public toilets, an illegal practice in many countries), cruising and visiting saunas, men can find many, even hundreds, of sexual partners – perhaps not all of them particularly choice encounters. From personal experience, women are a lot more selective about their sexual partners and it's hard to imagine a woman heading into a toilet and waiting in a darkened cubicle until a potential sexual partner walks in. Among lesbians, it's common to spend the night with the person, even on a one-night stand; whereas, with some men, as soon as the sexual act is over, the contact is finished, and one of them leaves immediately. It is not unusual for lesbians to spend periods without sex when they have no regular lover because the lesbian scene and community is not geared to finding sex in the same way as that of the men's community. Many lesbian relationships tend to be monogamous: sometimes women may even have the same sexual partner for life. While women desire exciting sex as much as men do, they often need some emotion behind the act, too.

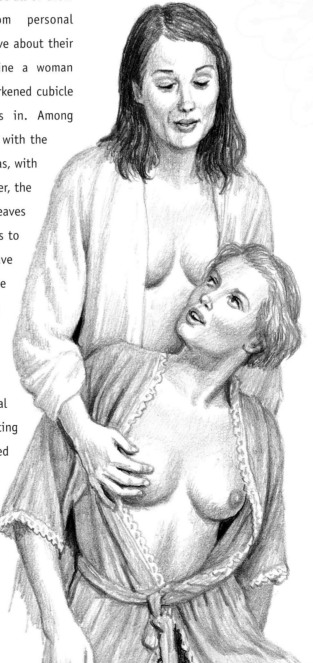

RIGHT Lesbians tend to have a different outlook on sexual encounters from gay men. While it is usual for a gay man on a one-night stand to leave directly after the act, it is not uncommon for women to spend the night together.

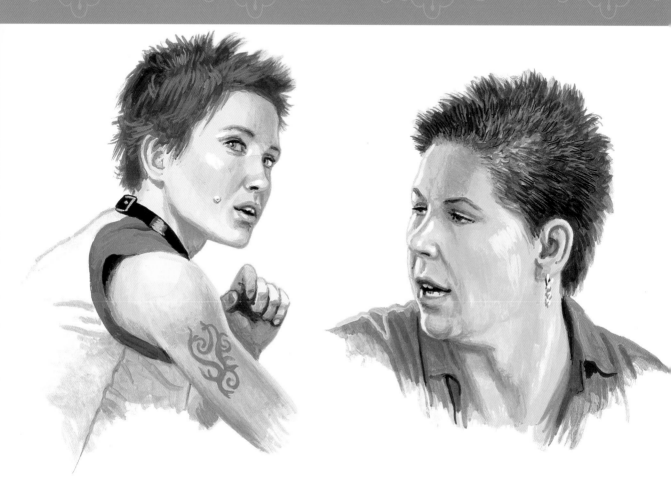

ABOVE Lesbians are a diverse community of people. A boyish trendy look, perhaps with spiked hair, good clothes and tattooing, is an increasingly popular and confident image cultivated among young lesbians, especially those 'on the scene'.

ABOVE RIGHT The 'butch' style is a common look on the lesbian scene. Women like their hair cut short and may wear baggier clothes, which do not show off the body. Butch women suffer from a great deal of stereotyping and prejudice, including the myth that they want to be men.

We also have quite a different response to sexual attraction. Gay male culture can be broken down into rigorous sexual types – young guys, hairy guys, gym bods, and so on – but the lesbian scene is not so vastly diverse. Nonetheless, we all have types of women we go for when we are looking for sex – young, older, boyish, feminine, butch, long-haired, short-haired, shaven-headed. But, unlike the gay scene, lesbian clubs do not tend to be as categorical as those frequented by many gay men.

Sexuality, though connected to our sex lives, is a different entity. It's what we are and not just who we sleep with, and it begins with 'coming out'. This is one of the biggest and hardest

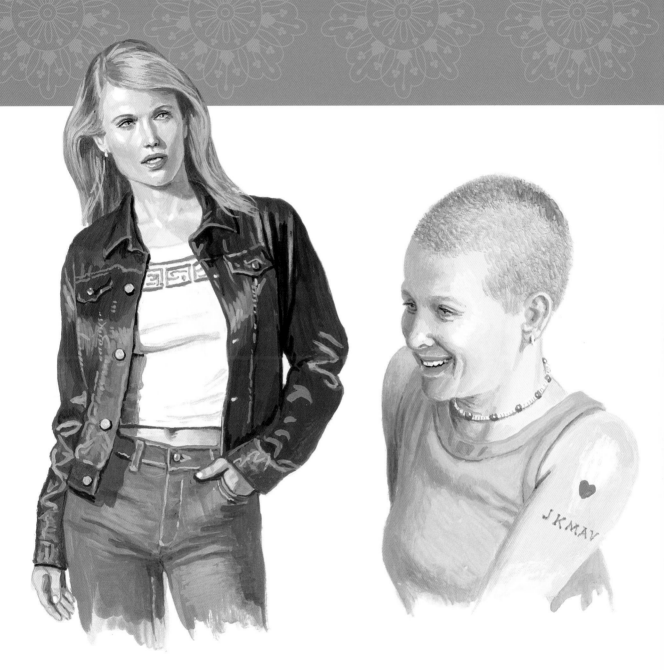

decisions to make. Though everyone you ask remembers how and when they came out as a lesbian, or even admitted that they were a woman who sleeps with other women, you realize later that this is just the first time you come out. You come out throughout your whole life, whether it's when you visit a doctor, a sexual health clinic, a financial adviser, or when you buy a lesbian magazine from the bookstore.

ABOVE LEFT Many women like the 'femme' look, with long hair, make-up and revealing clothes. Over the last decade these women became known as 'lipstick lesbians'.

ABOVE Lesbians tend to be daring in their appearance and many feel confident enough to choose a look that is not expected from women, including shaving off their hair.

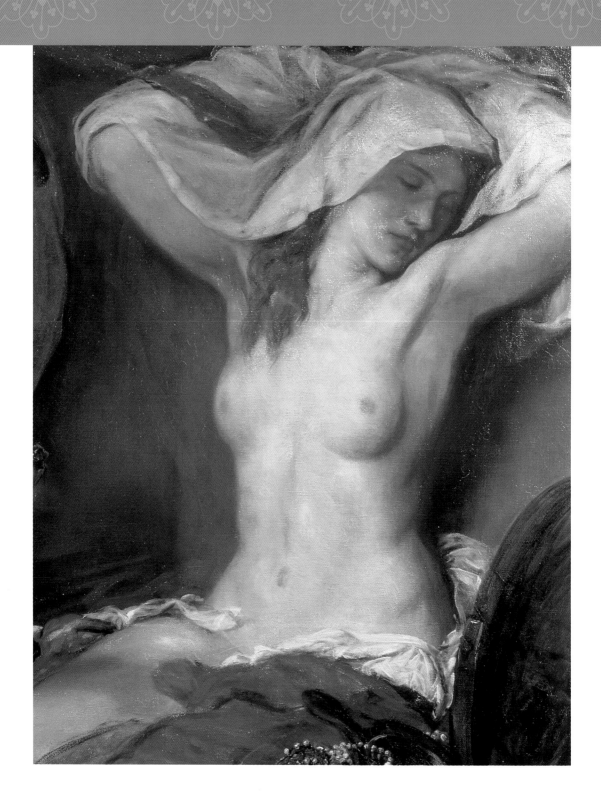

Emotional intimacy is another important part of lesbian sexuality. We tend to be relationship-orientated and this can create stereotypes. There's a famous joke that asks what lesbians bring on the second date – the answer is 'a removal truck'. Every one of us knows a friend or someone who immediately jumps out of one relationship into another and never spends time alone – the serial-relationship hunter. Relationships can be an important and fulfilling part of our sexuality, our chance to open our lives to someone else and to share what we have with them, emotionally and physically. Like sex, there's no right or wrong way to have a relationship: they can last two weeks or half a century. You may end up having many different relationships or settle for one life partner.

It is important, however, that the relationships you are in are rewarding, enriching and ideally give you a sense of fulfilment and equality. Some may be bad for you from the start, and the older and more experienced you get, the more you can recognize the signs and avoid potentially damaging involvements. Take comfort, though, because it's a rare woman who never made any mistakes when it comes to relationships. Almost all of us have one, if not more, ex partners we'd rather forget about.

The Kama Sutra holds the union of two people as an important physical and spiritual bond. It counsels us to experiment with erotic indulgence, but cautions that this should bring happiness as well as orgasms. Fusion of our bodies and our lives should bring perfect ecstasy and take happiness to another sphere. We should not only endeavour to make ourselves happy but also our partner or lover, too. To live in this way will make us appreciate the best things in life. It is then that our sex and sexuality are truly in harmony.

OPPOSITE 'The Amethyst Necklace', 1905, by Charles Haslewood Shannon (1863–1937). The Kama Sutra counsels lovers to experiment with sex, but it cautions that sex should bring more than orgasms. A spiritual bond makes the act of love more meaningful for both lovers.

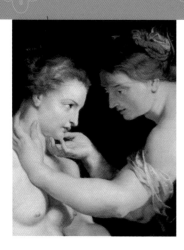

ABOVE Images of the Roman goddess, Diana, and her female attendants, among them her devotee Callisto, have been found on third- and fourth-century mosaic floors. Later, using Diana and her followers became a way of portraying titillating images of semi-clad women frolicking together without offending propriety.

Integrating our sexuality

As lesbians in Western society, we are in a better position than ever before to obtain happiness and stability, and we have more opportunities than women have previously enjoyed. It is only really in the last two decades that women have stopped coming under social and financial pressure to marry and the concept of the 'lesbian' has been born. Imagine your life if you had been attracted to women 100 or even 50 years ago. Unless you were independently wealthy, or in a position to be able to live a more unconventional lifestyle, it is highly unlikely that you would have been able to refuse to marry. For every Gertrude Stein or Radclyffe Hall who led an openly lesbian life, there were hundreds, even thousands, of other women who wanted to be in same-sex relationships yet ended up with husbands and children – and no way out.

Today lesbian women earn more money and lead independent lives. More and more of us feel comfortable coming out to family and friends, work colleagues and even doctors. We have access to services that never existed 20 years ago, such as sexual health clinics aimed exclusively at lesbians. We have greater access to a social life, and improved transport allows even those living in rural isolation to have easier access to lesbian venues. With most countries now having their own lesbian press, we can gain positive information and images of ourselves. This, and the advent of the Internet, has enabled us meet or talk about issues that affect and interest us. In fact, the Internet can even help us find partners.

We have the freedom to live together openly as couples, while many countries now allow us to register our partnerships; a few, such as Holland and Canada, even allow lesbian and gay couples to legally marry. Even five years ago this seemed almost impossible to imagine. We can affirm our love and relationships in front of family and friends and have them recognized by law. And we can adopt kids, or have biological children of our own, and raise them with our partners. The public profile of lesbians is growing, and there is a growing number of positive role models. High-profile entertainers, authors, musicians and television personalities feel able to come out, as do some professional sportswomen and politicians – again something unimaginable two decades ago. Every year, there are new and exciting opportunities; the quality of our lives is constantly improving, the recognition of ourselves and our relationships grows and we now have the chance, finally, to leave behind the subculture of secrecy, shame and insecurity which has imprisoned us until so very, very recently.

BELOW As lesbians we have more freedom that we did even three decades ago. We have greater access to a social life and more of us feel comfortable coming out about our sexuality and living openly together as couples.

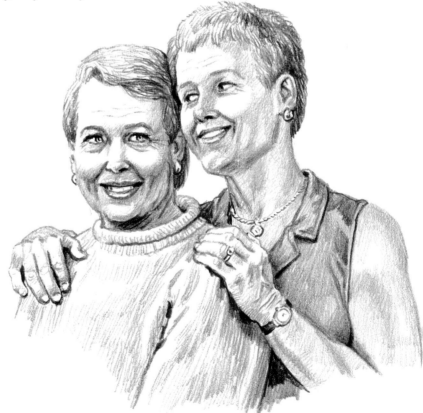

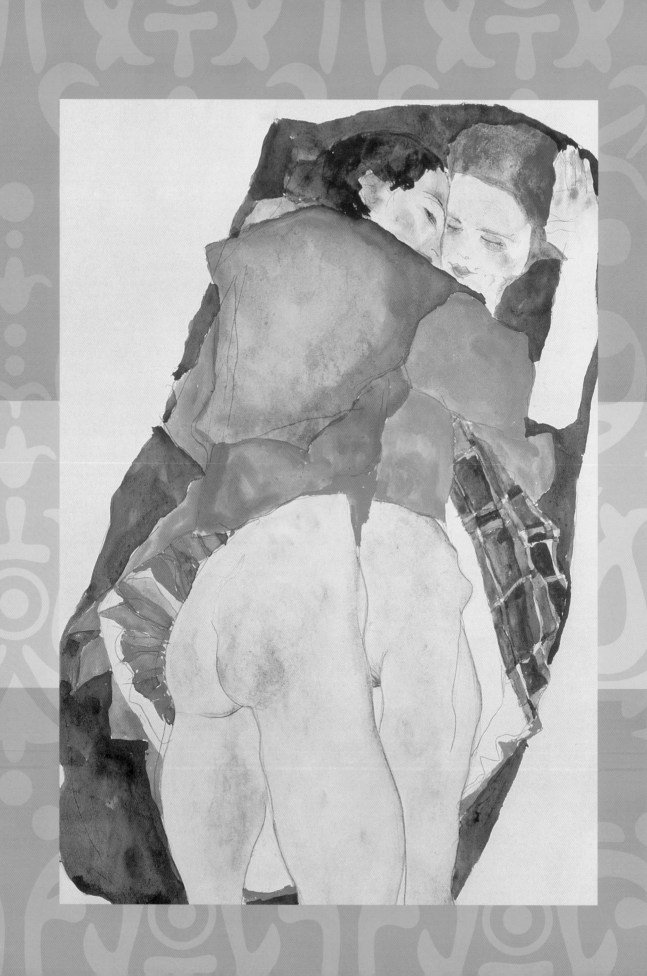

Chapter 3:
Preparing for love

sex and the female body

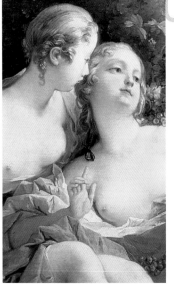

ABOVE One of the most important aspects of any relationship, especially a sexual one, is good communication between lovers. Without it we do not learn about each other and do not benefit from a lover's full potential.

OPPOSITE 'Embracing Couple' by Peter Paul Rubens (1577–1640). Greater awareness of our own bodies and sexual needs and wants will give us a better understanding of our lover's bodies and their sexual desires. Ultimately, such knowledge will make us good lovers.

Only in the last 30 years or so have women been able to speak openly, or read in magazines, about their sexual desires and needs. For lesbian women it has been a much shorter time.

Since the advent of our own magazines, books, sex manuals and porn videos we have been able to see and discuss our sexual realities, needs and desires. Lesbian sex is the coming together of two (or more) women in intimacy and pleasure. In a healthy sexual relationship, we should strive to please our partners or lovers with the same commitment and enthusiasm as we'd like them to show us. Therefore, by understanding our own bodies we can understand our lover's and, together, we can use the workings of our body to create pleasure for ourselves and the women we have sex with.

The clitoris

Fact: The female clitoris serves only one physical function – to give sexual pleasure. That's why it's the most important part of our physical sexual being. The clitoris contains around 8,000 densely concentrated nerve endings; the highest proportion in the body and twice the number found in the penis. Recent evidence suggests that 75 per cent of women require clitoral stimulation before reaching orgasm. This compares to less than 20 per cent of women who achieve a vaginal orgasm alone.

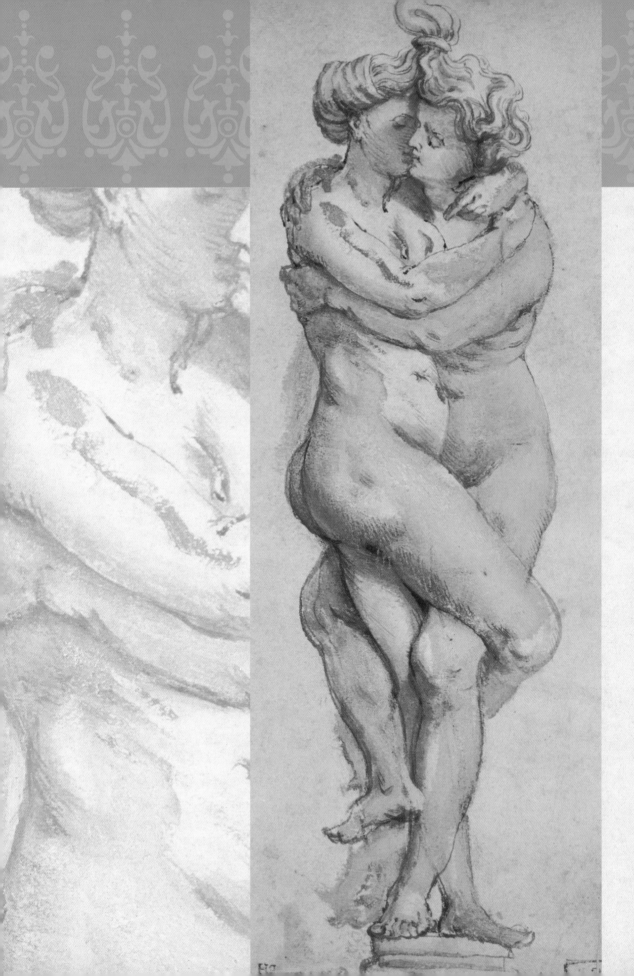

The clitoris, or 'clit', is the small nub of erectile tissue above the entrance to the vagina, which fills with blood and swells considerably when we become aroused or sexually stimulated. Only one part of it can be seen by the eye: the head, which is found beneath the clitoral hood. The clitoral shaft extends under the skin to the pubic bone and spreads into two arms – the crura – which extend around 7.5 cm (3 in) either side of the vaginal opening. One of the most sensitive parts of the female body, the clit is kept lubricated by oil-producing glands; this lubrication allows the hood to slide across the clit head with ease. Like all parts of the body, clits vary in size, colour and shape, and the head can be more prominent in some women. In others, the hood may cover the head almost completely, though this is unlikely to affect the ability to stimulate the clitoris. When aroused, the clit head gets bigger and the hood recedes slightly to enable better stimulation.

As clitorises themselves vary, so does each woman's individual stimulation needs. Some like firm pressure and need their clits rubbed hard to bring them to orgasm. Others enjoy a light touch or quick flicks, and find heavier pressure difficult to tolerate. A lot of women find nothing more exciting than having their clits licked or sucked by a lover's tongue or mouth; others find the sensation of a vibrator drives them wild. Women's clits also vary considerably in their responses after an orgasm. In some women, an orgasm makes them so sensitive that it takes a while before they can be touched here again. Others find that they can continue to be touched until they come again or, indeed, several more times. Women who enjoy multiple orgasms might find that the sensations become more heightened and intense with every orgasm; for others, however, the feelings decrease each time they come.

We all know that the clit is a wonderful part of the body, but it's only recently that medical science began research into sexual responses in women. In *The Sex Book*, Suzi Godson looks at research published in 1998 by Helen O'Connell, a urological surgeon in Melbourne, Australia, who discovered that clits were actually much bigger than was first believed. The nerve system, she discovered, went much deeper than just the clitoral head that was visible on the outside. An upside-down, V-shaped mass of erectile tissue, full of nerves and blood vessels, was found to extend from the clitoris into the body. This would certainly go some way towards explaining why an orgasm brings about sensations that transcend the vaginal area and go deep into the abdomen.

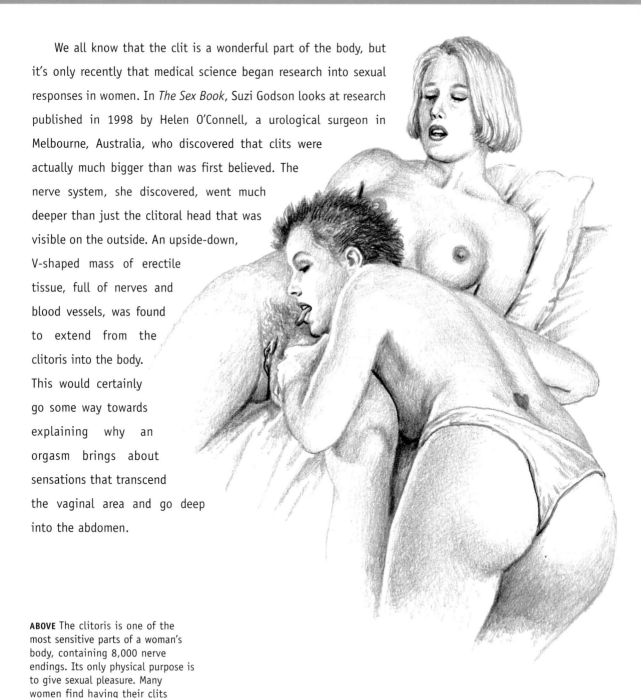

ABOVE The clitoris is one of the most sensitive parts of a woman's body, containing 8,000 nerve endings. Its only physical purpose is to give sexual pleasure. Many women find having their clits licked or sucked to be one of the most erotic experiences.

Outside the vaginal area

While the clit is the part of the body where we feel most of our sexual excitement, there are other parts of our vaginal areas, which may be equally erotic and can give intense pleasure. The external genitals, referred to as the 'vulva', include the outer lips (labia majora), the two, long folds of which are covered in hair and made up of fat and erectile tissue, and the smooth inner lips (labia minora) surrounding and protecting the urethral and vaginal openings. Inner labia vary enormously in women, perhaps more so than clits, because they are a larger part of the body and far more noticeable. Indeed, it's very common for both inner labia to be varying sizes and to find one lip hanging lower, or being of a different proportion from the other. This occurs in most women (so you're not alone) and is extremely unlikely to affect the sensitivity of that area. Some women have very small inner labia, which are hardly visible; others can be larger, sometimes protruding below the outer labia. Labia colour also varies from woman to woman, and can range from a light pink to dark brown.

When a woman becomes sexually aroused, both the inner and outer labia swell, becoming enlarged, which leaves the opening to the vagina more visible. The inner labia, which meet to form the clit's protective hood, also have a large number of nerve endings and play their own important part in sexual stimulation. Try tracing your finger away from the clitoris of your lover when she's turned on (or try this while masturbating). Slowly work your finger between the inner labia and notice the response you get or how you feel. This will be more sensitive when another person does it to you, or you to them, because neither of you is controlling your own movement or the pressure on your labia.

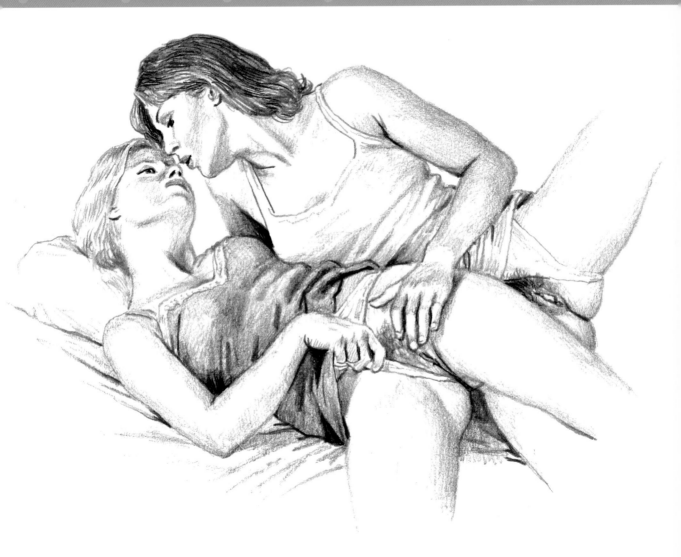

Another highly sexually charged area is the perineum. This is the flat line of skin starting at the base of the vulva, just under the vaginal opening, and extending back towards the anus. A soft touch with a finger, especially when the vagina is extremely wet, can produce highly intense feelings. Try wetting the area with extra lubrication, then tracing the finger along that stretch of skin, and watch for the response.

ABOVE We don't all enjoy the same things in sex, so exploring a lover is crucial in understanding what turns her on and what she likes.

Inside the vagina

The area inside the vaginal opening is also sensitive when touched or stimulated, though nowhere near as sensitive as the outer area. When unaroused, the walls of the vagina lie comfortably together. They absorb whatever is placed inside – the walls will form around a finger or dildo when inserted. The vagina's muscular tissue expands to accommodate whatever size object is inside the vaginal canal, whether it's a finger, sex toy or even a baby during childbirth. When a woman becomes sexually aroused, the rear part of the vagina extends and the cervix lifts, and this enables more comfortable penetration to take place. Since the internal vaginal area is less sensitive, it responds better to more vigorous and firmer stimulation, hence the need sometimes felt to have one or more fingers, a fist or sex toys used during penetration.

When it comes to care – keeping clean, healthy and lubricated – the tissue in the vaginal canal can be sensitive. It's advisable to avoid using soaps, detergents and toiletries which are harsh, chemical or highly perfumed as they can all lead to irritation and infection. Lubrication is important for the vagina and our sexual responses. The vagina lubricates itself all the time, though this increases hugely when one is turned on. Our ability to become wet is affected by a number of circumstances apart from arousal, including the hormonal changes experienced during adolescence, menstrual cycles and the menopause. Other factors affecting our natural lubrication include illness, and alcohol and drug use.

When we are aroused, the blood vessels inside the vagina become swollen with blood, the pressure of which pushes out droplets of fluid through the vaginal wall. These droplets come together and form a layer of silky, shiny lubricant that coats the vaginal walls. If you become aroused but don't have sex, the lubrication simply combines with your vagina's natural secretions and makes you more wet. While most women create sufficient lubrication for their sexual needs, some don't produce enough. How wet a woman gets should not be taken as an indication of how turned on she is; some women just naturally produce less lubricating fluid than others.

BELOW 'Bacchus and Erigone', by François Boucher (1703–70). Erigone, the virgin maiden, is associated with Bacchus, the bisexual god of wine, who extolled the virtues of hedonism and the pleasures of the flesh. Sex is a powerful emotion, but should ideally be about the joining together of body and mind.

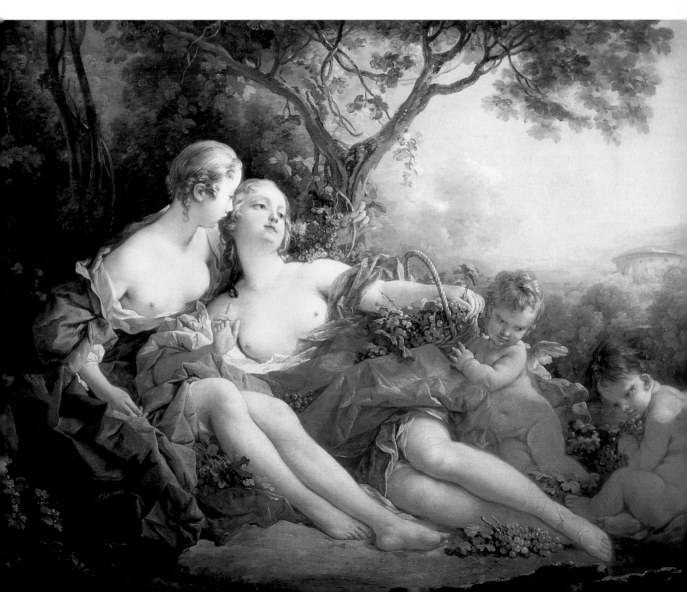

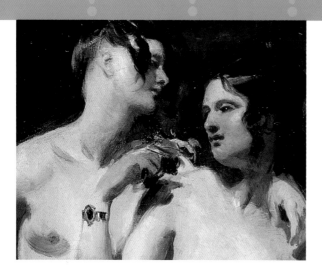

ABOVE 'Two Female Nudes' by William Etty (1787–1849). Touching your lover's body will be a hugely pleasurable experience for her. Ask her to tell you where her most sensitive areas are, or experiment with new erogenous zones.

Extra lubrication

Adding lubrication to your lovemaking sessions will help to make the whole genital area feel more sensitive and it can enhance the feelings and stimulation of the clit, inner labia and vaginal opening. The wetter the inside of your own or your lover's vagina, the easier and less uncomfortable penetration becomes (it causes less friction on sensitive skin). Although you and your lover might feel you are wet enough during sex, the use of artificial lubricant can add another dimension to the sexual experience. Although women can be a little offended when you bring out a bottle of lube during sex, this soon dissipates when you cover their whole vulva in lube, and they experience the intense sensations that come from the slippery wetness on their already wet vaginal areas. On an aroused woman this area normally gets quite hot and the lubrication tends to be much cooler. When you touch a hot vulva with lube, the sensation of just a slight temperature change can prove a huge turn-on, as can the feeling of rubbing your wet vagina against your equally wet lover.

These days, there are large numbers of lubes available, including water-based, silicone and glycerine-based. Visit a lesbian and gay-friendly sex shop, or check out mail order sites on the Internet to find the whole available range because pharmacies might sell a limited supply. Water-based varieties tend to be safest, being largely taste-, smell- and stain-free (although you will notice a taste the first few times before you get used to it). They also tend to irritate the genitals less than any other types and wash out easily after sex. The other advantage of this kind of lubricant is that if it dries out during sex, a small amount of water (keep a small glass by the bed) will reactivate it on the vagina. It does tend to dry out on the skin, making it unsuitable for skin massage.

Check out the ingredients and try, where possible, to avoid any lubes containing a substance called nonoxynol-9. It's a spermicide that causes genital irritation, as can the substances methyl- or propyl-paraben. Women with yeast infections should avoid glycerine-based varieties. Test lubes on the wrist to check for any adverse reaction before the moment of passion.

Lubes can also be highly beneficial for women during menopause, who find they don't get as wet as they used to during sexual activity. They should also be compulsory for anal play, anal sex or vaginal fisting (see pages 99, 105, 109–10). The anal canal produces no natural lubrication, so it can tear or be damaged by inserting even a finger (imagine, then, an unlubricated sex toy!). When it comes to fisting – inserting a fist into the vagina – you might feel you don't need as much lube, especially if whoever is being fisted is very wet. Both the hand and vagina should be well lubricated; it helps for a smoother penetration and minimizes any risk of damage during the insertion or removal of the fist. Avoid substances such as massage oils or petroleum jelly because they don't wash out of the body easily. They can also rot latex items, including dental dams, condoms and gloves and, therefore, are hopeless for safe sex (see also pages 133–5). The use of lubrication is not for everyone; maybe some of you have tried it and find it makes you too wet or less sensitive However I would certainly advise trying it either on your own or, even better, with a lover before you decide you don't want to use it.

Breasts

Another important component of the female physical and sexual make-up is the breasts. Like our clits, labia and vaginas, breasts are unique to every woman. They come in all sizes and shapes, and also in all levels of sensitivity. It is not uncommon for some women not to like having their breasts played with or even touched, while others can find their breasts and nipples so sensitive that they can orgasm from their stimulation alone. In between these two extremes come the women who like to have their breasts caressed or their nipples pinched or flicked as a foreplay to, or during, clitoral/vaginal sex. Some women prefer to have their breasts fondled or stroked tenderly, others like them touched a lot less gently before having their nipples played with.

There are many ways to pleasure a lover using her breasts – kissing, biting them gently, kneading one in your hand, rubbing your breasts against hers. The breasts can be sensitive and, after a certain amount of play, your lover might say she doesn't want you to continue. Progress from her breasts down her belly, perhaps with your tongue, playing along the contours of her body until you reach her vaginal area and begin stimulating there.

While some women don't enjoy having their nipples touched, others adore it. Women who have very sensitive nipples may only be capable of a small amount of play. Rubbing the nipples (even through a bra) is a good place to begin, and unless they're already erect, you'll feel them harden to your touch. Gauge your lover's response and, after a while, if she's enjoying what you are doing, begin pinching them (again, some women like gentle or moderate pinching whereas others prefer it hard), or roll them between your finger and thumb. Having your nipples licked or sucked can be highly erotic, especially when your lover teases – flicking a tongue over one and then moving away to the other. Playing with each other's breasts at the same time is also a fulfilling act during foreplay and can be a big turn-on.

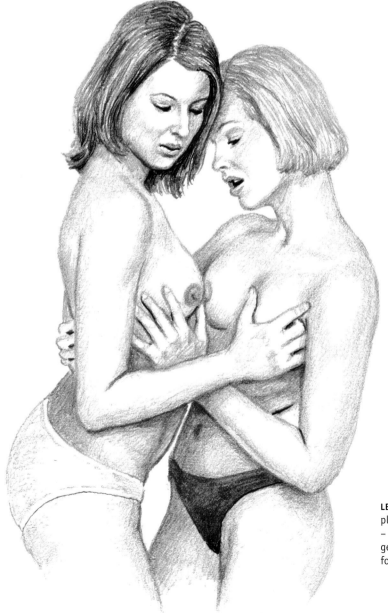

LEFT There are many ways to pleasure a lover using her breasts – kissing, biting or kneading them gently can all prove a big turn on for her, and you.

Seduction and foreplay

There is only one time when foreplay is not an important part of sex and that's when you're both so turned on and desperate to satisfy each other that the idea of foreplay seems an annoying digression. When we first meet a woman we want, the sexual need is urgent and our desires constantly simmer beneath the surface. We can't keep our hands off each other, and tend to spend most of our time turned on and ready for sex.

However, as the intense feelings mellow, or your relationship grows, foreplay becomes an important part of sexual expression. It's an opportunity for wonderful exploration of the entirety of your lover's body and sexual needs, and she can get to know you and your wants. Foreplay can be any number of things, from body language, touch and massage, kissing and embracing to love talk.

BELOW Foreplay is an important part of sex, preparing both women mentally and physically for the act of love. Touching or kissing is a good way to get intimate with a lover.

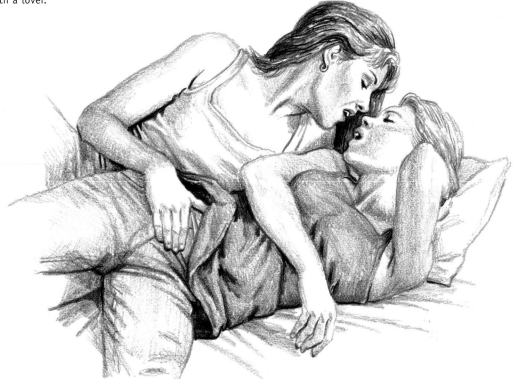

You're out, you see a woman and you're attracted to her. Perhaps you'd like to become closer to her, get to know her a little better, take her out on a date or even take her home that night. But is she attracted to you? Will she be interested or will you make a fool of yourself if you approach her? While there are no hard and fast rules about seduction because every woman is different and behaves in her own unique way, there are certain signs to watch for. When you see someone you like, make eye contact. If they're looking at you, glance away and then look back; if they're still looking, the chances are that they're at least curious. See who she's with and if she looks as though she's obviously with a lover, steer clear unless you are interested in the possibility of making friends (but even then, exercise a great deal of caution because you don't want to end up in trouble).

Rejection can hurt, so if you want to approach her, it's best not to do it in front of all her friends, or even yours, if you're not entirely certain of the response you'll get. Wait until she's alone at the bar and go up and say hello. Begin chatting casually, and if she looks like she's responding, continue the conversation. If she's

ABOVE Seducing someone else or being seduced by another is an exciting experience. Find out what she likes by gauging her response to what you do to her body.

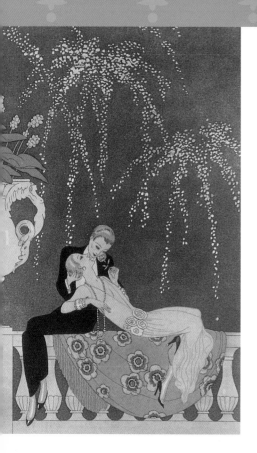

ABOVE 'Fireworks', a 1925
lithograph by George Barbier.
You can normally tell if someone
is interested in you through
eye contact or body language.
Learning how to read the signs
will help you to avoid rejection.

disinterested, distracted or wildly looking around for her friends,
you should probably try to find someone else.

If she's interested in you, it will eventually become apparent.
She might look you straight in the eyes or shyly flirt with you via
eye contact. A person who is sexually interested in another will
usually give the message away through the eyes, and the pupils will
dilate when someone is turned on or feeling sexual attraction. Look
at how she is holding her body and listen to what she is saying.
Check whether these two elements match up or are contradictory.
Is her body turned in order to be close to you? Is she watching the
moves you make, perhaps even mirroring them – for example, when
you take a sip of your drink, does she do the same? Does she listen
intently to what you say? If you give her your phone number and
she doesn't ask for yours, she may want to get to know you better
(you'll know if she calls), but if she asks for your number, she's
definitely interested.

It's easier to find women who might be sexually interested
in you in a lesbian bar or group, but what about in a non-gay
environment, when it's not so easy to make your intentions known
or to be blatant in your flirting? Here, you will need to be more
circumspect. Check her body language for signs she's interested
(see above, pages 64–5 and 114–18). She, too, may be treading
carefully in a non-lesbian environment, and she might not be too
comfortable giving out physical signals. Talk to her, and then throw
in some questions. Ask her what books she likes, mention a few
lesbian authors and ask if she's read anything by them, or question
her about lesbian films. If she is interested in you, then she, too,
will be dropping hints in the hope of gauging your reaction to her
questions. If she's not giving off blatant signals, ask her out for a

casual coffee. If she says no or makes an excuse, then you'll know she's not interested; if she says yes, then you will have some time to find out more about her.

Rejection happens to us all at some time or another and maybe that encounter, relationship or person wasn't meant to be. She might be rejecting you because she already has a partner or lover, she may not want to have casual sex, she could even be straight or just plain not interested. And yes, getting turned down does hurt, but it's best not to take it too personally or let it affect your self-worth. When you feel ready, you can always try again with someone else, and the next time might be the right time.

BELOW It's easiest to find women who might be interested in you in a lesbian bar or group, but in a non-gay environment it may not be so easy to flirt openly or make your intentions known.

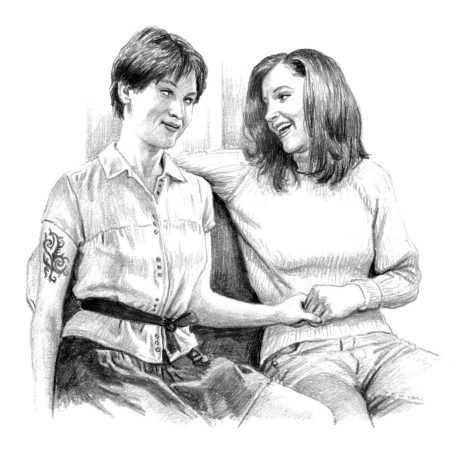

Body language

BELOW Understanding body language can help you to work out if someone is interested in you, and whether it is worth pursuing them. Take note of a woman's casual touches, facial expressions and the proximity of her body to yours as you talk.

There are many ways to become intimate with your lover as a prelude to the sexual act. Body language, one of the skills the original Kama Sutra says should be studied, is just one aspect of physical attraction. It's an important form of expression because, with practise, it enables one woman to understand the intentions, moods and motivations of another. Body language is a psychology that can be applied in many situations, whether you are meeting someone for the first time or in a long-term relationship.

When meeting a potential sexual partner for the first time or communicating with a lover, a smile or eye contact can be revealing and intimate. A smile is the sign of universal friendliness and reassurance, but most people can tell whether it's genuine or not. Not meeting someone's eye, looking away during conversation or looking directly into the eyes of a lover or potential lover all send out crucial messages about behaviour, intention and desire.

Physical proximity and closeness are also important aspects of body language and usually a signal that increased sexual intimacy is desired. Moving closer to a person with whom you would like to get intimate can give you an idea of whether they would like to do the same with you. If they move back to create more space, you can assume that they're not interested; if they don't move away

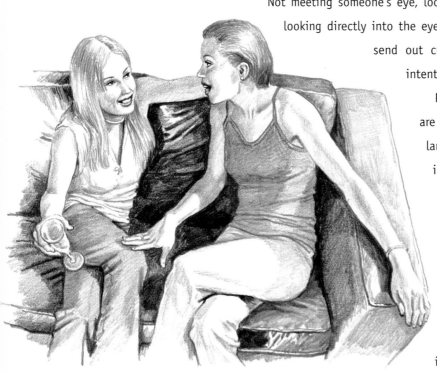

or, perhaps, even turn their body towards you and move closer, it is safe to assume that they would like to become more intimate. Body language can be easier to interpret with a long-term lover because you have more knowledge about each other's subtle movements and know each other's signals. You understand their dislikes and how they behave when they desire sexual closeness and intimacy or want to avoid it.

BELOW A 'Shunga' (erotic) print from 'The Island of Women' *c* 1870. In a group of women, physical proximity is important, because it is a signal that increased sexual intimacy is desired. Moving into a woman's personal space will indicate that you want to get close.

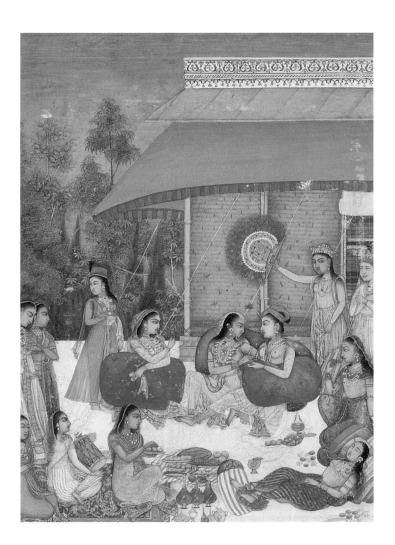

Kissing

The Kama Sutra also places a high importance on kissing as a part of foreplay and one of the first stages of lovemaking. It's an extremely intimate act and again gives both lovers a wonderful opportunity for mutual exploration. The manual looks at the different types of kissing at each stage, from seduction to the sexual act itself and afterwards. It goes from lip-brushing to tender little kisses which lightly touch the lover's skin, eyes, neck or cheeks, to the more passionate kisses, deep and hard, where lovers explore each other's mouths with their tongues; this is called 'the soul kiss'. As passion mounts, the lovers urgently probe each other's mouths, and the tongues then come together in the 'bliss kiss'.

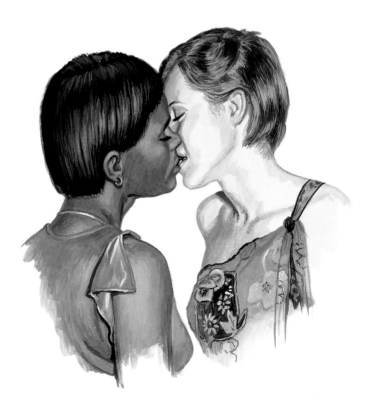

RIGHT Kissing a lover is an intimate act. Although it looks simple, it requires a certain amount of skill if it's to be done well – like many other aspects of sex.

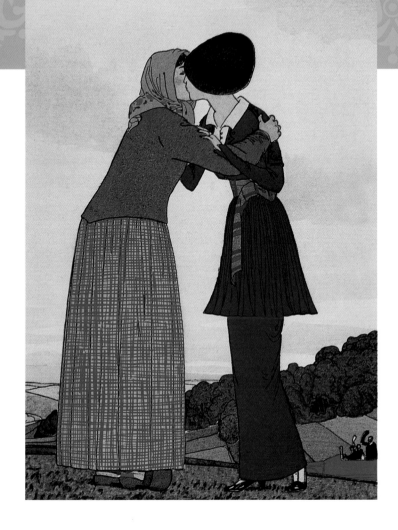

LEFT 'Gazette du Bon Ton', a costume plate from 'Les Soeurs de Lait, robe d'après-midi de Doeuillet', showing two ladies embracing, by Andre-Edouard Marty (1882–1974). Kissing someone for the first time can be perfect but sometimes you might need practise to get it right.

Sucking the tongue of your lover very gently can also be a highly erotic experience, as can slipping in just the tip. The lips, like the genitals, contain nerve endings and swell with blood when we kiss someone we sexually desire. Women kiss in many ways; each of us prefers different methods and techniques. Although it looks simple, kissing, like other aspects of sex, requires a certain skill. Sometimes kissing someone for the first time can feel perfect; at other times, the 'choreography' between the two of you might need some practise. It's very rare that two people are completely incompatible when it comes to kissing, but it does happen and perhaps the chemistry between you isn't quite right after all.

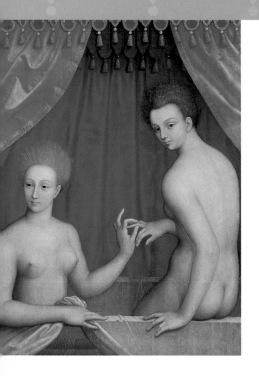

ABOVE 'Ladies Bathing', c 1500s, by the Fontainebleau School. Even the slightest touch, as long as it is done properly and in the right place on the body, can send a lover wild with desire.

OPPOSITE Scratching a lover's skin is an intense act. Run your nails along her shoulders, breasts, down her belly and to her thighs, and watch her response.

Touch

Of all the erotic senses, touch is the most important and it can convey a wide variety of nuances to both partners. The touch on the hand, arm or thigh can be as much a part of the flirting process as eye contact or a gorgeous smile. When you're filled with sexual longing for someone, that first touch or even that 'accidentally on purpose' brush of hands can send sensations racing straight to the clit. Holding hands is an important part of a relationship and brings with it closeness for any two people. While it's an intimate act, it can serve to be sexual, or even offer reassurance. The hand is also very likely to be one of the first parts of your lover's body you will touch, so it has great significance.

While we all think about the breasts, nipples, clit and labia as being the sexual parts of the body, the skin itself can be treated as one big sex organ. Sensitive and responsive, it's the foundation for all erogenous zones, and touching it can bring incredible, wonderful sensations. Even the slightest brush of your fingers across her neck or shoulders, or running one finger down the curve of her back can drive some woman wild. Something as small as tracing in between your lover's fingers with one of your own can be deeply erotic, especially when your finger is wet. Also, try sucking your lover's fingertips.

Scratching and biting your lover before, and during, sex can be extremely arousing, and both activities are detailed in the Kama Sutra. Like all touch, it can be light and gentle, or vigorous and rough. Some women enjoy soft bites to the neck, shoulders, inner thighs, nipples and breasts. Try a bite combined with the sucking of the skin; it'll leave a small bruised area – a love bite or 'hickie'. Some women can get very aroused from the pain of being bitten.

The key is to start off lightly, then make it harder if that is what she wants. While you might get carried away in the pleasure, be aware of each other's safety and limitations.

Scratching also varies in intensity and one should be careful not to be rough to the point where blood is drawn (unless this is wanted by one or either woman, but even then the scratches should be properly cleaned afterwards). The act of scratching a lover's skin is an intense one, and watching their response can be a turn-on for you. Gently, or firmly if that's what is desired, scratch your fingernails from her shoulders, across her breasts and even nipples, down the belly, thighs and legs and then back again, perhaps stopping at her vagina on the way back. Watch for her response. Light, gentle caresses will inevitably lead to more intense and fervent touches.

The Kama Sutra emphasizes the rubbing and pressing of the body in amorous acts with another. Rubbing skin with your lover is another crucial part of foreplay that can prove extremely intense and sensual. Rubbing the genital areas together, or where one aroused woman rubs her vagina over the thigh of her lover, can be deeply pleasurable. Sometimes, there's nothing sexier than feeling another woman's breasts, with her nipples erect, rub slowly along the length of your back – or vice versa. Even more intense is the feeling of your breasts, covered in massage oil, sliding very slowly from her oiled pubic area along her stomach up to her breasts, where you then circle them with your own.

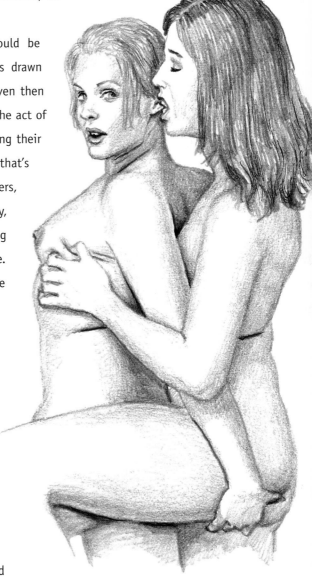

BELOW Just touching your lover can be a huge turn on, especially when both women know the most sensitive parts of each other's bodies, such as their nipples or breasts.

Every touch of a body provides both the person doing the touching and the receiver with different sensations, and anything you try is a great exercise in getting to know your lover's sensitivity tolerance, likes and dislikes.

Pressing, meanwhile, conjures up an image of something more urgent. The act of pressing bodies against each other, or pressing your partner's body against the wall, hips thrusting into one another, can give a delicious, wild feeling to both women, especially if this is being done outside or in a place where sex is either hurried or furtive. When clothes separate you from your lover's skin, that, too, can be an exciting part of foreplay. As your tension mounts and you explore her body by rubbing your hands over her clothes, you'll both find that a hand thrust inside the jeans or exposing a breast in order that you may tease or lick the nipple can be highly exciting. It gives you both an idea of the delicious sex that lies ahead when you finally get to have it.

BELOW Having clothes separate you from a lover's body can be erotic and tantalizing, and make sex even more exciting, especially if it's furtive or hurried.

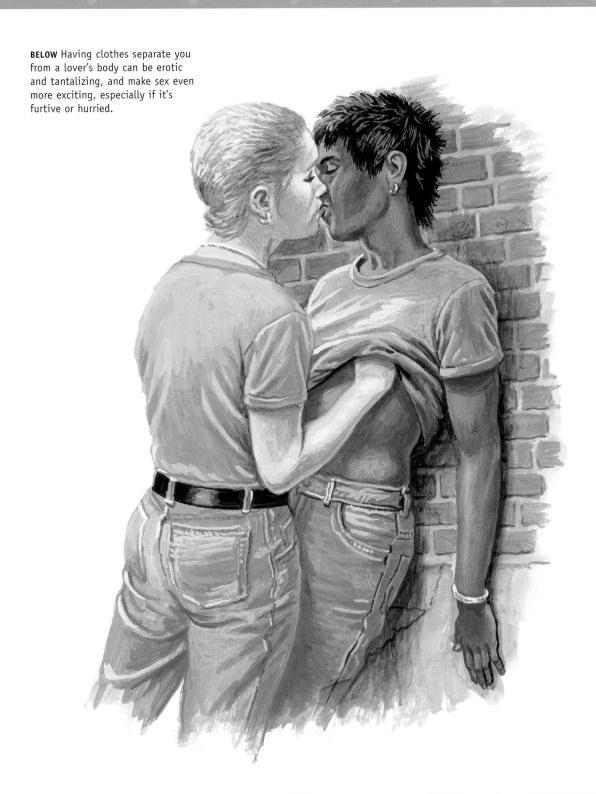

Love talk

Making noise and love talk is an important part of the sexual experience for some people. Even the slightest noises can bring about large responses in a lover. Groans, moans or grunts during sex and especially during orgasm can make some women feel they are coming, too. Others enjoy being talked to or like to 'talk dirty' during sex, and derive a lot of pleasure from telling a lover – or being told – what is going to happen to them. Some women are quiet during lovemaking and prefer to make almost no noise at all, but whether you are noisy or quiet, neither means you're the better lover. The only problem that can arise is if you get embarrassed by the noise levels your lover makes, or she becomes a little insecure if you don't make noise, making her think she's not satisfying you. This is where communication is crucial. Sometimes, when the mood is right, it can be wonderful to moan your head off, but, similarly, deliberately keeping quiet and directing your vocal energies into your orgasmic energies can be just as intensive and sexy.

Getting close to a lover

You can have sex with someone and not be emotionally close to them. Sometimes you can be attracted to someone, want sex and an orgasm, and that's all there is to it, simple as that. Getting close to a lover, whether casual or long-term, requires open and honest communication and a desire to confide in that particular person. At the root of this is the acceptance that just because we are with another woman, it does not mean we're the same. We've already seen that our bodies differ vastly from woman to woman, as do our sexual and emotional needs. Sometimes we might like the same thing as our lover, but more often than not, we enjoy different

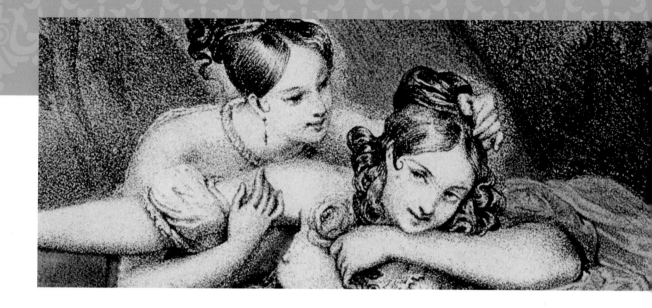

touches, sensations and activities. If those elements are very different, then we might find we're not sexually compatible. But, on the whole, differences can make relationships stronger and the sexual experience more intense and varied.

The essence of the Kama Sutra is the open and honest exploration of sexuality and our own desires. Therefore, it's important for us to be honest with ourselves about what we like and not to be embarrassed or too shy to ask for it from a lover. Similarly, it's equally important to be honest about the times we don't want to have sex, even if a lover does. It might be disappointing for them, but it will be worse if one of you feels pressured into having sex when you don't want to – that's a guaranteed way of creating resentment. There will be times when we want sex desperately, and other occasions when our sex drives are low. It's then that communication is most important, so that one lover can reassure the other. Communication is a two-way process and, to be effective, it requires that our lovers or partners are equally honest about how they feel. It's only through honesty that we can develop trust in each other and, with trust, we can experiment more and work at helping each other push our boundaries further in the exploration of our sexual selves.

ABOVE A whisper in the ear in 'Adam, Do Be Quiet', *c* 1830, by Victor Adam. Some women like to have a lover talk to them during sex. If you don't feel confident in talking dirty, just telling a lover what you would like to do to her can be enough.

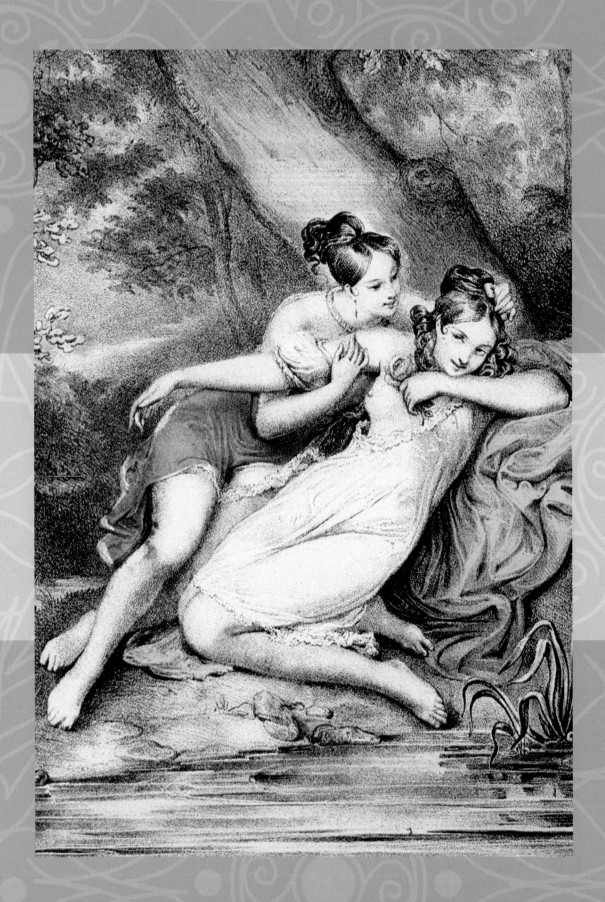

Chapter 4:
On making love

self-masturbation

Successful and satisfying lovemaking
relies as much on imagination as
it does on skill. Understanding, and
experimenting with, your own desires
is the first step towards becoming a
considerate, sensuous and skilled lover.

'Playing with yourself', 'self-love', 'solo sex' – whatever you prefer
to call it, masturbation plays an important part in our sexual
development and is not, as myth would have it, something we do
when we can't get – or aren't having – any sex. In fact, it's the best
way to learn what you like sexually.

Research from the Kinsey Institute at Indiana University in the
USA showed that 70 per cent of women who were interviewed
admitted to masturbating. Yet, while we might talk about sex with
friends, how often do we discuss masturbation? Admitting that we
masturbate is a big 'no'. Since the beginning of time, humans have
touched their genitals for enjoyment. As very young kids we do it
because it feels nice, though masturbating for sexual pleasure
usually begins with puberty. Some women, however, may not start
to masturbate until later in life, when they have shed the
inhibitions or fears they experienced in their youth, while others
may not ever masturbate at all.

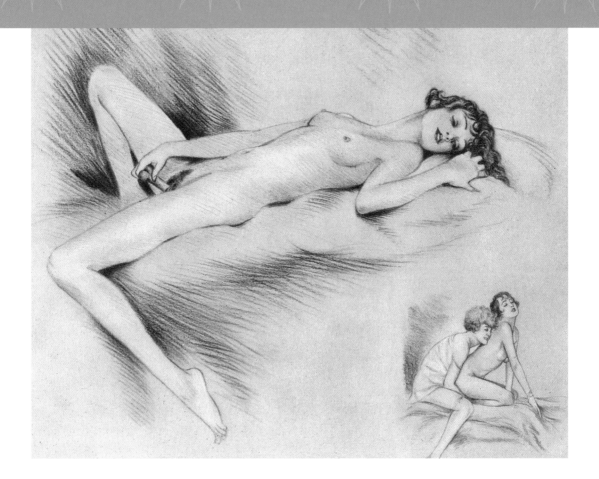

Sadly, this innocent and pleasurable pastime, enjoyed the world over, is still much maligned. In the past, masturbation was seen as a pathological perversion. Even now, despite the fact that women's magazines, and lesbian magazines in particular, talk about female masturbation, it is rare to find a woman who has been taught from an early age that masturbating is good. Rather, as kids and teens, we get told that it's bad for us, even wrong, which can leave us with feelings of guilt or shame. In fact, it wasn't until 1972 that the American Medical Association pronounced it a normal sexual activity. The shame is that we get these negative influences when we're at our most sexually confused and inexperienced – during adolescence.

BELOW Masturbating is the perfect way to learn what you enjoy sexually and how your body responds to different stimuli, whether using your hand or a sex toy.

Most of us learn how to masturbate through trial and error. By experimenting as we go along, we find a technique that works for us and we stick with it, or vary it according to our sexual development or life circumstances. There are no right and wrong ways when it comes to methods or the amount of times we masturbate because we all like different techniques and need varying levels of stimulation to achieve sexual pleasure and orgasm. Some women masturbate frequently, even daily, others only occasionally.

Masturbation techniques

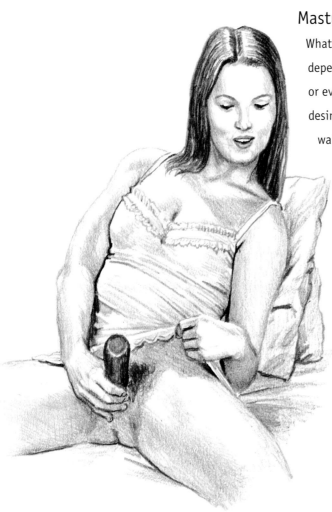

What we want from masturbation often varies, depending on such variables as the mood we are in or even what time of day it is. Sometimes you might desire a quick orgasm before going to sleep or on waking up in the morning; at other times, you may want to take your time and really enjoy what you're doing, making masturbation a pleasurable whole-body experience in which you can experiment with different techniques, sensations and materials – touching and caressing your breasts, nipples and thighs, dressed or undressed.

The most common technique is to lie on your back or stomach and, using one finger or more, rub the clit either from side to side or stroke it up and down. The pressure of the stroke depends on you and what you like. It can range from firm or hard rubbing, tracing your fingers back and forth between your labia, or lightly brushing the head of the clit. Experiment with a variety of strokes and pressures to experience different responses within your body. Try using lube during masturbation to add extra sensitivity (see pages 56–7).

Every woman masturbates in her own way. Some like to stand up and find they get a different sensation from the orgasm than they would have had if they were lying down. Using fabric to masturbate is also very common. This is where women get extra stimulation from the friction of material against their clits by either rubbing themselves through their underwear or with a blanket, sheet, pillow or duvet. Other women receive a lot of satisfaction from rubbing up against objects when they are dressed – perhaps resting the clitoral area on a table corner and rubbing against a hard surface. Take care when rubbing the clitoris with a material: doing this too vigorously can cause soreness or even abrasions from the friction. Some women get pleasure from rubbing or pressing their thighs together, exerting pressure on the clit through squeezing their muscles.

Water is another fun way of masturbating, especially where a showerhead is used to direct a powerful spray on the clitoris and vagina (never aim water directly up the vagina and make sure it's not too hot because it can burn).

Many women like penetration while they masturbate and insert a finger (or fingers) or a vibrator or dildo. For greater sensitivity, cover your fingers or the toy you are using with lubrication. It is not uncommon for some women to want anal stimulation while they masturbate, inserting a finger or butt plug – a mini dildo that is inserted into the anus. (Never put anything that has been in the anus in the vagina as this can pass on bacterial infection.)

Masturbation is the safest way to push your own boundaries and experiment with techniques and your own sexual response. If you've never tried it, then get a mirror, preferably one you can lean against a wall so as to leave both hands free, and watch yourself masturbating. Notice how, the more turned on you get, your clitoris and vagina change colour and become engorged. Study your physical response to using different toys on yourself and, if you can, watch how your genital area reacts when you orgasm. Masturbation is a fun exercise by which you learn about the workings of your body, its sexual arousal and release.

The key to good masturbation is relaxation; you need to let yourself go and you can't do that if you're not at ease with yourself. Try relaxing in a warm bath or using soft lights and gentle music. Privacy is also important, especially where you share a living space with someone else, including a partner or lover. And if we have a partner, it's normal to still want to masturbate. Sometimes a lover might want you to watch them masturbate and a lot of women find this an extreme turn-on, but it's not disloyal to prefer the privacy to be alone with your own thoughts and fantasies.

Many women who find it hard to orgasm with a lover can do so easily during masturbation. These women should, therefore, practise masturbation first to gain confidence in their sexuality before expecting orgasms from sex with a partner. Learning to pleasure yourself is important because once you know what you like and how to make yourself come, then you can teach your lover what exactly turns you on. Get her to be open with you too and find out what makes her hot. When women know how to masturbate well, they are normally knowledgeable enough to be able to pleasure a lover well, and it's a rare for a person not to want to be a good lover.

Mutual masturbation

Stimulating each other's clits – otherwise known as mutual masturbation – plays an important role in lesbian sex. Touching your lover while she touches you can be highly exciting. Don't be afraid to experiment with new things together, particularly if you are lovers who have been together for a while. If you are in a long-term relationship, you'll find communication is just as important as it is when you have sex with someone for the first time. Does she want you to stimulate her clit hard, or does she like it to be done gently? Does she enjoy you teasing her labia? When you communicate your desires clearly (and this applies to all aspects of intimacy), the sex just gets better and better. Just because you already know someone sexually, this doesn't mean they want the same lovemaking time and again. If your lover likes to be rubbed hard and fast, maybe you should try rubbing her very slowly, tracing back and forth along the hood of her clit, paying attention to her clit head with small movements and bringing her to orgasm in a different way. If you're having sex for the first time with a particular woman, then it's probably best to ask her directly what she enjoys, rather than rely upon guesswork and experimentation – which can come if you have sex with her again. Mutual masturbation with a lover is always exciting because it offers a vast and exciting number of possible positions.

BELOW Communication between a couple is important when it comes to mutual masturbation because what you like may not be enjoyable for your partner. Asking her directly how she wants to be touched is usually the best approach.

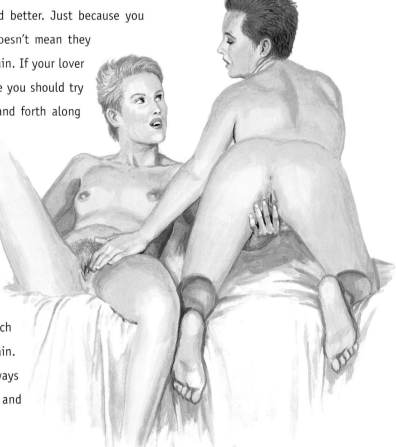

RIGHT Everyone has a particular position they prefer and from which they get the most sexual satisfaction. Experimenting with different techniques is a good way for lovers to become comfortable with each other.

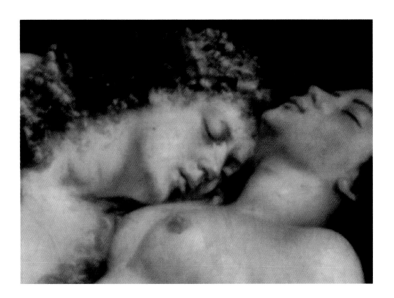

Side by side

With an arm round each other, this position gives each woman easy access to the other's clit. Using the forefinger to stimulate the clitoris enables the index finger or the remaining fingers to penetrate and stimulate your lover's vagina.

Kneeling face-to-face

This position also gives both women easy access to their lover's clit. In fact, kneeling provides better access and allows each lover to have both hands free. So, while you stimulate your lover and she stimulates you, you can play with each other's breasts, pinch and tease the nipples, trace your hands across her buttocks, scratch up and down her back or even penetrate her (vaginally or anally with toys or fingers). One of the sexiest things about this position is the fact that it enables you to watch your lover as she plays with you, or you with her. Maintaining eye contact during sex is a highly intimate act and it also allows you to watch her face as she comes.

Standing face-to-face

This position allows couples to kiss, press or rub their breasts together and achieve full-body contact. It gives you a free hand to play with your lover's body or to penetrate her. Standing face to face also allows you both to put a thigh between each other's legs and exert pressure on the genitals while both clits are being stimulated. Feeling a wet, aroused vagina on your thigh while you are being stimulated is a huge turn-on. This position is very intimate, and it allows both women to get extremely close in order to stimulate each other. It also enables you to watch your lover as you touch her.

Standing back-to-front

Here, one woman faces away from her lover. The woman behind stimulates the clit of the lover in front and can insert the remaining fingers of the same hand or a sex toy inside her partner's vagina. With her free hand, she can hold her lover's waist or give attention to her breasts or nipples. Meanwhile, the lover in front can reach back and simultaneously play with the clit of the other woman.

Spoons

This position allows very close bodily contact. Both lovers lie on their sides, one in front of the other; the one behind reaches an arm over the side and to the vaginal area of the woman in front, while the other reaches back to her lover's clit. Feeling pubic hair, the aroused vagina and even thrusting movements of your lover's hips against you can be very exciting. This position, however, doesn't make it easy for either partner to use their free hand to stimulate each other's bodies. Spoons is a gentle way to make love, perhaps if you're tired or after a long session of lovemaking.

The female orgasm

An orgasm is the release of sexual tension built up in the body during stimulation. It is a series of involuntary and intensely pleasurable contractions that involve the pubococcygues, the powerful muscle that helps to support the pelvic floor. While the feeling can be experienced in the genitals, the perineum and even in the rectum, an orgasm is more than merely a genital pleasure. When the body orgasms, the pleasure waves and contractions extend throughout the body, from the head to the feet.

For different women, orgasms can take many forms. In fact, our own orgasms may vary every time we experience them and can depend on a number of things – where we are, how aroused we are, even what is being done to us. Sometimes, they can be deep and intense; at other times, the sensation of an orgasm can be considerably less powerful than you expect. As I have said earlier, there are many kinds of orgasm and debates over the decades have primarily concentrated on clitoral and vaginal orgasms. In the last couple of decades, the G-spot orgasm has also been introduced as a concept (see pages 89–90).

Fact: Almost all women who achieve orgasm do so through clitoral stimulation, rather than through vaginal penetration, and even when a woman has a vaginal orgasm, it is common for her to have had her clit stimulated beforehand. Vaginal orgasms usually require thrusting pressure from whatever penetrates the vagina – fingers, dildo or a fist – and for the woman being penetrated to be very aroused. Where clitoral orgasms seem sharper and more intense, vaginal orgasms feel as though they come from deeper inside the body. It isn't uncommon to get confused as to where your orgasm is coming from, especially if you're aroused and being penetrated while having your clit stimulated. You experience all kinds of pleasurable sensations – the sharp intensity of a clit orgasm and the deep throbbing of a vaginal orgasm at the same time.

Multiple orgasms

Not all women experience multiple orgasms. Some have all the sexual satisfaction they need after one orgasm, and find their clits are too sensitive to come again. Others may feel responsive enough to enjoy continuous stimulation, even after orgasm and will come again and then feel satisfied. And it's not uncommon for some women to require continued stimulation even after they've come several times. The intensity of climax experienced during multiple orgasms varies considerably from woman to woman. Some find the more often they come, the weaker their orgasms become, whereas in others the sensations get stronger and become more intense with every orgasm.

How much time needs to pass between orgasm and continued stimulation also varies considerably, as can the time that passes between orgasms. It might be that after the first orgasm, a woman may want a couple of minutes before her clit is directly touched again, while others come and can continue to have their clits stimulated straightaway. If you're very turned on during sex and you come quickly, it may take a while to orgasm again, whereas some women can orgasm and, within minutes, are coming again.

Techniques for multiple orgasms

Women who experience multiple orgasms while masturbating sometimes find that they are unable to do so with a lover. Some people are naturally multi-orgasmic but if you haven't enjoyed a

BELOW Every orgasm we have can
be unique from the last one we
experienced. An orgasm from
clitoral stimulation – by a finger or
toy – can feel very different from
one achieved by penetration.

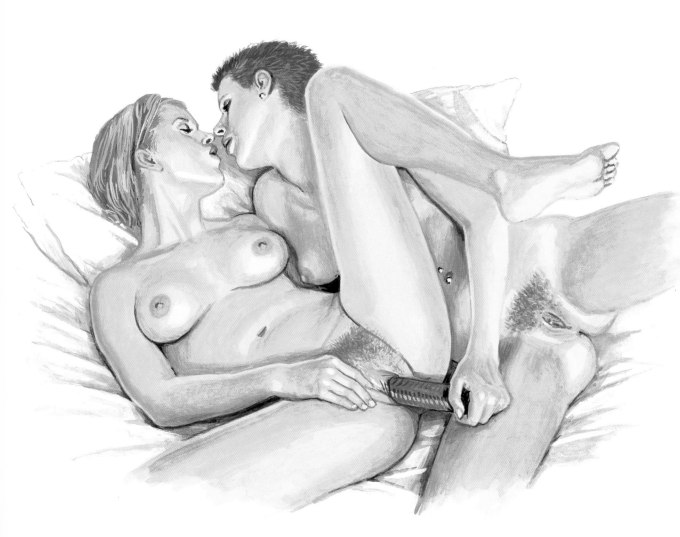

multiple orgasm so far, this doesn't mean you won't be capable of coming several times. Lovemaking requires patience and practise. The best way to learn is through masturbation. Once you've had an orgasm, continue stimulating yourself to see if you can attain another. Some women find that they can keep stimulating their clits after orgasm, but if you haven't experienced multiple orgasms, it's very unlikely that you will be able to bear having your clit touched at this stage.

If you find your clit is oversensitive, change where and how you stimulate yourself. Use some lubrication (see pages 56–7), if you aren't already wet. If you have become a little dry from the friction of rubbing your clit, that dryness will heighten your sensitivity and make your clitoris more difficult to touch. Touch your vulva and maybe trace your finger along the length of your labia, avoiding the clit head. Using your natural wetness or lube, gently touch around the base of your clit and, after a while, move up and down at the sides of your clit hood, a side at a time. After a certain amount of time, you should be able to start touching the clit hood again, perhaps slowly at first before increasing the pressure and speed again. Your clit will let you know exactly when it's ready to start being directly stimulated and so enable you to bring yourself to orgasm again. If you want to continue, practise again after your orgasm. The better you get to know your post-orgasmic responses, the more often you'll be able to come.

If you're practising with a lover, tell her exactly what you want. Encourage her to try giving you different kinds of orgasms, perhaps with her fingers or a vibrator the first time. Then she can use her tongue to bring you to the second orgasm (or vaginal for the first and clitoral for the second). Only you know what's right.

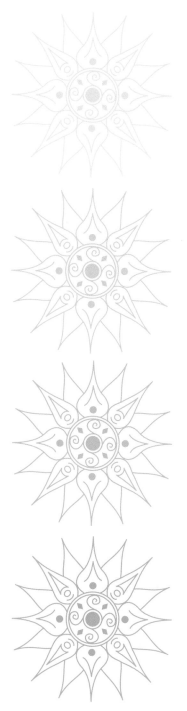

Simultaneous orgasm

When you come at the same time as your lover, it's a great turn-on for both of you. More often than not, though, it's more by accident than design. The best thing to do is not to try too hard because it puts you and your partner under pressure. Instead, practise reaching simultaneous orgasm together first. Lovers who know each other's sexual responses can usually tell when their partner is about to come. While you are stimulating her, watch for her response. If you see she's getting too aroused and could soon orgasm when you aren't ready, stop touching her. The timing is crucial here because there are two stages to pre-orgasm – near to orgasm and about to orgasm. Near to orgasm is when the waves are building up and you know an orgasm will come, but you can still stop if you want to; about to orgasm is that point where you are going to come and there's no way you can prevent yourself. If stimulation stops too soon – or altogether just before climax – the orgasm can lose its impact and intensity. So, if your lover is in that near state and you know it's not too late, stop stimulating her (or vice versa, if it's happening to you). The partner who needs more time can continue to be stimulated until she nears orgasm. At this point, the waiting partner should be stimulated again and hopefully the timing will be right.

Delaying orgasm

Not only does delaying an orgasm make your orgasm (and that of your partner) more intense, but it can also lengthen arousal and the actual sex act. Practise on your own during masturbation and see how many times you can bring yourself to the brink before you come. As I mentioned earlier, simultaneous orgasm is as much down to chance as it is to skill. Not everyone can have a multiple orgasm or come at the same time as their lover and everyone has different physical needs. While orgasms play an important part in our sexual experience, sometimes one partner might be more orgasmic than the other and need to climax more before feeling sexually satisfied. Often, bringing a lover to climax can be pleasure enough. In fact, making a woman come while restraining yourself can be very sexy.

The G-spot

The term 'G-spot' made its way into popular culture in the early 1980s with the publication of Whipple and Perry's *The G-Spot and Other Recent Discoveries about Human Sexuality*. The name comes from German gynaecologist, Ernest Grafenberg, whose research in the 1950s led him to the discovery of an area inside the vagina which, when stimulated, could lead to an orgasm or ejaculation. Whether it really exists, or it's just a sexual response in certain women, is open to question. Certainly, some women think it does exist and that its stimulation can result in an ejaculation of fluid and an intense orgasm. Others are confused by its physical location. There is a danger in seeing the G-spot as an all-important sexual button, just waiting to be pressed. This can make some women feel disappointed or inadequate, especially if their lover ejaculates and they don't.

ABOVE Bringing yourself to the brink of orgasm and stopping before you actually come requires discipline. Try it a few times and you'll see how intense your orgasm is when you finally allow yourself to come.

The G-spot is the small, spongy mass of tissue (about 4–5 cm/1½–2 in long) wrapped around the urethra. It can be stimulated through the vaginal wall with fingers or a sex toy. While we may all have this urethral sponge, everyone responds to stimulation differently. Pushing at the urethral sponge will just bother your bladder if you aren't sufficiently aroused. Practise finding your G-spot during masturbation. Lie on your stomach and when you're about to come, place a finger or two into your vagina and press them against the front wall, searching for a spongy, more sensitive area. Sexual arousal makes it easier to find your G-spot but because of its physical proximity to the bladder, stimulation of this area can make you feel as though you want to go to the bathroom. It's natural and after a while, the feeling will go. See if you can bring yourself to orgasm. For those determined to find it, buy curved dildos or vibrators, which place pressure on the spot.

BELOW An eighteenth-century 'Shunga' woodblock of two women making love by Koryisai. Some women can achieve orgasm by the stimulation of their breasts alone.

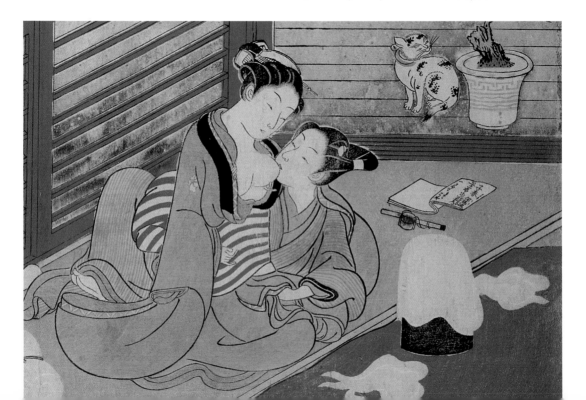

Female ejaculation

No one quite knows what it is, or why some women ejaculate when they come, while others don't. The ejaculate comes from the urethra, normally when a woman orgasms, and is generally associated with stimulation of the G-spot. Women can ejaculate from intense clitoral stimulation – perhaps after stimulation has gone on for a long period of time or if stimulation continues after one orgasm and up to the next.

The ejaculate fluid is much thinner and more watery than the substance that comes from men. In some, the fluid shoots from the vagina, particularly during penetration by a fist (see page 99). But in other women, the fluid will just flow and flow from them and can leave a bed particularly wet. Women who sometimes ejaculate liken the sensation to that of having a pee, though the fluid itself isn't urine. Because it's not a common occurrence, women who ejaculate, especially with a new lover, can sometimes find it embarrassing although it's impossible to prevent an ejaculation when it happens. It's best to explain to a partner that it could happen before making love for the first time, so that your partner is aware. A lover ejaculating over her arm or onto the bed could come as a shock.

For some women, ejaculating can be an emotional experience, especially when it happens during orgasm, because there is a feeling of complete and utter physical release – fluid and muscle together. Ejaculating can be a wonderful thing, but not all women do it. In fact, most women don't, so there's nothing wrong with you if you're one of them. With practise it might happen for you, but if it doesn't, it's not meant to be and you should certainly still aim to get as much pleasure as you can out of trying other new things, alone or with a partner.

Oral sex

There are a number of expressions: 'going down' and 'eating pussy' are just two of those commonly used. Whatever term you prefer, it means the same thing: cunnilingus – oral sex on another woman. The term comes from Latin *cunnus* meaning 'vulva' and *lingere*, 'to lick'. But oral sex means a lot more than just licking; it can refer to sucking or nuzzling the clitoris, labia and vagina of your lover, often bringing her to an intense orgasm. It is a beautiful and passionate way for lovers to explore each other physically and mentally, and to find out what it is that you both enjoy.

While going down on someone is an important part of lesbian sex, some women will be a lot more shy about letting or asking their lover to lick and suck them because they are self-conscious about the smell of their vaginas. Just as our clits and labia are different, so are the smells and tastes of every woman's vaginal area. The taste, in particular, can change at various times of the month – a woman who is a day or so away from getting her period will taste quite different (the vaginal juices are slightly more bitter) from the way she'll taste during ovulation. Whether it's you or your lover, who's a bit reticent, introduce a shower or bath into foreplay. It's a great way of getting close to each other and should also make you feel more confident if you feel you're clean.

Good oral sex requires both lovers to take their time and relax. Women need different amounts of time to get fully aroused and eventually orgasm. If your lover takes a while, you have to be prepared for that, so don't start too vigorously. Build up the pressure and speed, perhaps picking up in the few minutes before she orgasms. (Be warned: Over-vigorous oral exertion can cut that little web of skin under your tongue – it heals in a couple of days.)

Instead of just starting at the clit – unless that's what she wants – pay attention to the opening of the labia. Trace it with your finger or work your tongue along the outer lips, kissing the entrance or gently flicking the tip of your tongue into the vaginal opening before you open or get her to open herself fully for you.

Opening up the labia will reveal beautiful, soft, moist flesh, which can vary in shades from pink to brown depending on the individual. You can gently penetrate her with a couple of fingers before moving your tongue along the inner labia and up to the clit. Using your tongue, touch the tip of the clit and flick it gently or stroke it across the top. Some women like light, quick continuous strokes on their clit; others prefer to be licked in a firm, rhythmic way, finding a light touch too sensitive or ticklish. Note how your lover responds. Some women enjoy being teased so you can lick around the clit, maybe missing the most sensitive part, or every now and again coming back and licking across the top when your lover least expects it. As your speed and pressure increases, so then you can increase the intensity of the thrusting movements if you are penetrating her. If your partner wants a deeper penetration, insert a well-lubricated dildo inside her (see pages 108–9).

Another technique involves drawing the flat of your tongue across the length of her vulva and labia, dragging it as slowly as possible all the way up to her clit, perhaps stopping there to suck it instead of licking. Some women adore having their labia

BELOW Lick or suck your partner's clit, teasing, playing and varying the pressure and quickness to judge her responses.

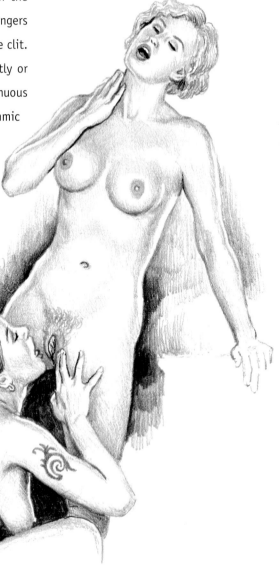

BELOW The 'sitting on the face' position is one of many that allows for penetration at the same time as oral sex. Combining both can often give a woman a mind-blowing orgasm.

sucked, finding it as arousing as clitoral stimulation. Each woman responds differently and what worked in the past with one lover might be the same with the woman you're now going down on, so communication is crucial. Remember, it takes time to learn about an individual woman's desires and needs, so don't worry about it all being perfect – there's plenty of time.

Face between thighs

This is the most common of positions. One lover lies on her back with her legs open, while her partner lies down between her legs with her face in the vaginal area. This gives good access to the clit and also enables vaginal penetration with fingers or sex toys. Use the other hand to play with her nipples. For multi-penetration, insert a thumb in her vagina and a finger in her anus. This position can also be varied, whereby a partner kneels between her lover's legs, or where one partner sits in a chair and the other woman kneels in front of her.

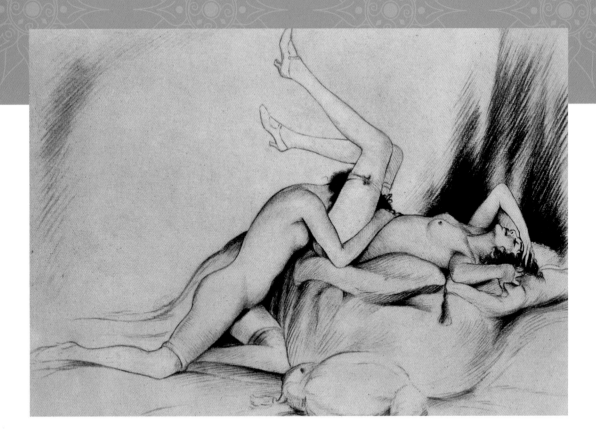

Sitting on the face

Here, one lover kneels over the face of her lover who is lying beneath her and lowers herself down onto her partner's waiting mouth. The partner below can stimulate the clit with her tongue and reach up to the nipples of her lover. This position also allows penetration either by fingers or with a dildo.

Standing–kneeling position

One woman stands with her legs slightly spread, while her partner kneels in front of her and stretches her face and tongue up to the vaginal area and clit above her. The standing partner might want to lean against the wall for support, especially if she takes a while to come, because standing in this position can be tiring over a long period. Similarly, the partner beneath might need a pillow, if she's on the floor. Stimulating a clit by tongue in this position can provide a different sensation from having it stimulated when lying down.

ABOVE An illustration from Eugène Reunier's 1920s 'Tower of Love' lithograph series depicting a variation on the 'face between the thighs' position.

'Sixty-nine'

This is the most famous of oral sex positions and sometimes the most difficult to perform well. Here, you and a partner lie down, one on top of the other, with one's head facing the vaginal area of the other. This is not the easiest of positions because women's physiques vary. The one lying down will require pillows to lift her head (you'll need support for the neck, otherwise you'll be craning to reach your lover's vulva). The lover on top then kneels over her partner's face and extends her body down to her vaginal area.

Make sure the heavier partner is on the bottom and that it's easy for you both to breathe. Another version of this can be done where you lie side by side, again facing in opposite directions. However, this doesn't give such easy access to the vaginal area and can prove more restrictive.

BELOW In the 'Sixty-nine' position, it is only too easy to sit back and enjoy the sensations you are experiencing, rather than to put effort into the act. But done with skill and some concentration, this position can be fulfilling for both women.

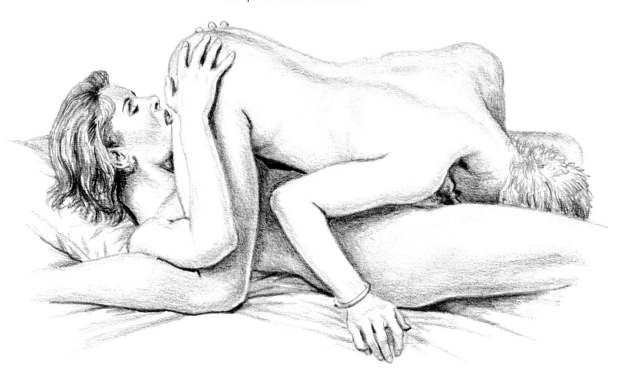

Penetration

Some women don't like penetration, or don't feel a need for it; others adore it. Like everything else, we're all different, and if you don't enjoy penetration, there's nothing wrong with that. Women who like penetration have different preferences; some are satisfied when a finger or two is inserted (usually while they have their clit played with), others prefer a deeper penetration and like to use sex toys or be fisted (see below). Some like the penetration to be gentle, sometimes not even thrusting too much at all – often, the sensation of having the vagina filled is enough, while others enjoy a vigorous and fast thrust. The elasticity of the vagina accommodates childbirth, so the vaginal canal will expand to accommodate accordingly. Also, capacity for what you or your lover want inside can change, depending on how aroused you are. The more turned on you are, the more likely it is that you can accommodate more and take more vigorous stimulation. And the more your vagina gets used to being penetrated, the easier it is to have more sizeable objects inserted, moving from fingers to toys, then changing the size of toys.

There are a variety of ways to penetrate, and angles you can use, and all of them have their own sensation. If your lover is lying on her back, it's usually easier to reach deeper inside her, back towards the cervix (some like the sensation of fingers behind there – others can find it painful). Or reach to the front to find her G-spot, the spongy mass behind the pubic bone (for more detail, see pages 89–90). Penetration is one of the most versatile of activities and there are a lot of options – standing, sitting, lying on your back or stomach, kneeling, squatting or bending over an object like a bed or table. Penetration can take place while performing oral sex and even simultaneous anal stimulation, if your lover likes that (with some coordination, all three can be done at the same time).

Penetration can be a wonderful sexual experience, but care should be taken. Don't insert anything too big to begin with. Let the one being penetrated decide what size works – you might find that you like something smaller inside you while your lover prefers a bigger toy. You can always build up to bigger toys if you require a fuller, deeper penetration. Be careful about inserting objects, making sure there no sharp or rough edges. Similarly, be sure fingernails are smooth and well trimmed; jagged or long nails can cause cuts, scratches and bruises inside the vagina. While the vagina can take a great deal of thrusting and may accommodate toys and fists of all sizes, it is still very sensitive and can easily be damaged. Play responsibly and don't get into dangerous situations.

LEFT Some women only like a finger or two inside them during lovemaking, while others want deeper and more vigorous penetration, preferring a lover to use a dildo or vibrator for a stronger sensation.

Fisting

This is where one partner inserts her whole hand inside her lover's vagina. The lover performing the fisting must take time and care over the act. Hand size obviously plays a part in the act; the smaller the hand, the easier access should be. First, to insert a fist requires a lot of lubrication and whoever is getting fisted needs to be relaxed and very turned-on – otherwise, the fist will not go in.

A well-lubed latex glove can make entry easier because it's much smoother than skin. It's best to start by inserting a couple of fingers as far they can go, building up to all four fingers. When all four fingers are in, tuck in your thumb as far as it goes in your palm. The widest part of your hand is the area at the base of the fingers and this is the hardest part to get in, so it might help to cup your hand slightly, perhaps squeezing your fingers together to lessen the width. If it hurts your partner too much, stop immediately. But if the pain is pleasurable and she's happy to continue, keep pushing very slowly until the hand finally enters. When it does, curl your fingers around your thumb and form a perfect fist or, if she prefers, leave your fingers slightly uncurled so that you can get access to the different areas inside her. The thrusting pressure and movement should be very gentle when you are fisting because over-enthusiasm could cause damage.

BELOW An orgasm achieved from fisting can be very intense but when it's happened, the vagina can close itself around the fist, so withdraw very slowly, taking utmost care.

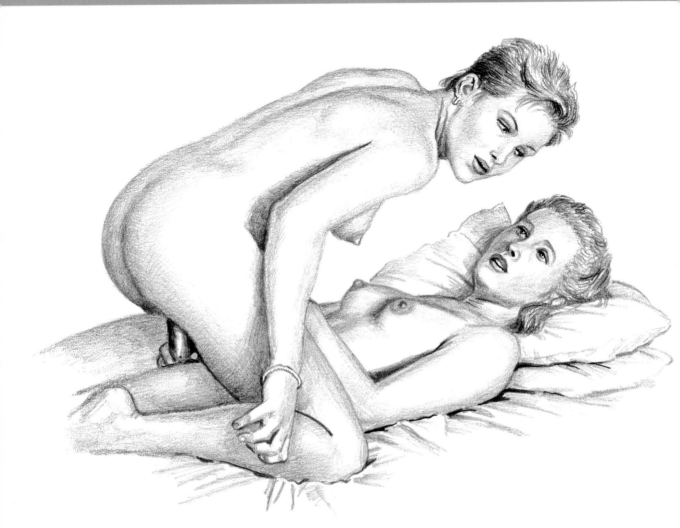

ABOVE Having a lover penetrate you while you sit on top of them allows for a dildo or vibrator to get deep inside you. It also gives you greater control in both the speed and depth of movement.

Front-to-front position

This is the most common of penetrative positions. Here, the partner on top (either with a hand, or a dildo in the hand or worn in a strap-on harness) penetrates the vagina of her lover beneath. With all penetrative positions, there can be an advantage to wearing a dildo in a harness as it leaves both hands free for clitoral stimulation and to play with the nipples and breasts. It also enables partners to remain close during sex and kiss.

The pelvic lift

Here, one woman lies on the floor and her partner kneels very close between her legs. The lover underneath lifts her buttocks up from the floor and is supported on the legs of her kneeling partner. This works better when the partner on top is wearing a harness as it allows them both to have hands free to give better support to the partner underneath.

Knees-to-chest position

This is good for deep penetration. One woman lies on her back and pulls her legs up to her shoulders (this requires agility), exposing her vaginal entrance and clitoris to the lover in front of her. If the position becomes tiring, the lover with her legs up can rest them against the shoulders of her partner. The penetration, however, is not as deep when this slight change happens. A variation of this can be done where just one leg is lifted. This, too, allows for very deep penetration.

BELOW Using a dildo in a harness can sometimes be the best method, as it frees up the hands of the lover who is doing the penetrating. She can add to her lover's sensations by playing with her clit or teasing her nipples.

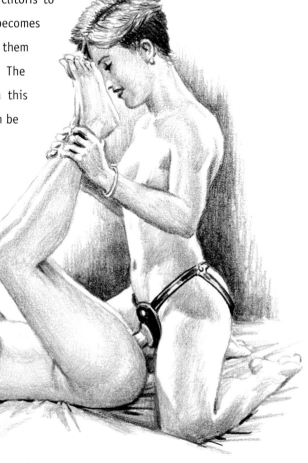

Sitting on top

One partner lies down with a harness and well-lubed dildo. The other partner then lowers herself onto it; the one below thrusts upwards as the one on top thrusts down. Both partners can play with each other's breasts and nipples while the woman on top can play with, or have her partner play with, her clit. This position does require a lot of strength, especially from the partner underneath, but allows for deep penetration. In a variation of the position, the partner on top faces the other way and stimulates both her own clit and the clit of the woman underneath.

Double-penetration

One lover lies down and the other lies between her legs. Both are vagina-to-vagina and a double-ended dildo is inserted into both vaginas. Although this doesn't allow for a lot of movement, it does make the sensations rather intense and allows each partner to stimulate her own clit.

Sitting on a chair

The heavier partner should be on the bottom. Here, one woman sits on a chair without arms. With her fingers or a dildo (in or out of a harness), she penetrates the woman who sits astride her, facing her. The partner below can stimulate the clit of the partner above or play with, or nuzzle, her nipples. Meanwhile, the woman on top thrusts downwards, while her partner grinds or thrusts upwards. This position requires some leg strength from the partner underneath. As a variation, the woman on top can also sit facing away from her partner. This allows both lovers to thrust more deeply in the same direction and can stimulate the G-spot.

From behind

This position enables a lot of stimulation and deep penetration. One lover kneels on all fours, while her partner kneels close behind. She can penetrate with her fingers, or with a hand-held dildo, leaving her other hand free to play with the clit or nipples of her partner. With a harness, she has the freedom to play with the clit and the nipples simultaneously. For a deeper thrust, she can hold onto one shoulder, while stimulating the clit of her lover. Curved dildos and vibrators are available for the purpose of stimulating the G-spot.

As a variation, the partner underneath is bent over an object, like a table or the back of a chair. Another popular position is where one partner leans on a low object, say a coffee table, while her standing lover penetrates from behind.

BELOW Penetration from behind can result in very intense orgasms. The position allows for deep penetration and stimulation of the clit at the same time and can feel a little more dominant than face-to-face lovemaking.

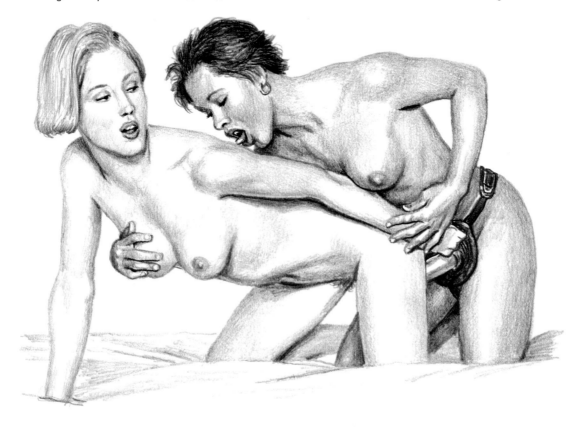

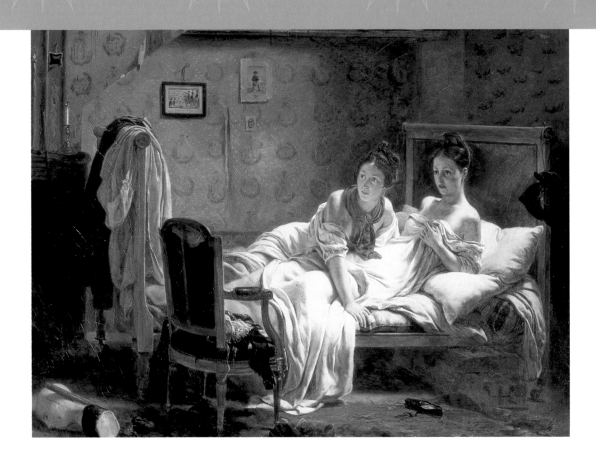

ABOVE 'Two Women in Bed' by
J A Rohne, *c* 1800s. We all have
our boundaries and it's important
for us to respect our lover's limits.
Respect is as much a part of good
sex as technique, and a woman
should never be cajoled into doing
something she doesn't want to do.

Standing position

When both lovers are standing, it allows each woman to penetrate
the other. Two or three fingers can be inserted and the thumb may
be used to stimulate the clit. Similarly, hand-held dildos are easy
to insert, which allows women to keep stimulating each other's clit.
Where one woman is penetrating the other with a strap-on dildo,
the woman being penetrated might want to lean back against a wall
for support. Similarly, one lover can penetrate her lover from
behind with fingers or dildo, while stimulating her clit. For the
woman being penetrated, the sensation of her naked flesh against
the cold wall and the hot flesh of the woman behind, thrusting into
her, can be a huge turn-on.

Anal sex

Some women find anal sex a highly pleasurable activity; others can't even bear the idea of it. The anus has a great number of nerve endings, which make it highly sensitive. It can also be a very arousing part of the body if it is stimulated in the right way, particularly if it's done with clitoral stimulation or vaginal penetration (or both). Anilingus – or rimming – is where one partner licks at the opening of the other's anus. Slow, circular movements can prove unbearably sensuous. However, the receiving partner must be clean and it's advisable that some form of latex barrier is used between tongue and anal entrance.

Anal penetration can be done after rimming to increase pleasure, but it can also form a complementary part of your lovemaking. If your partner is happy with the idea, and it has been discussed beforehand, slip in a finger while you are stimulating her vagina – the smallest pressure can drive some women wild, while others can take more substantial penetration. Always talk about it first – it may not be the kind of surprise your lover will appreciate. Always use a lot of lube if engaging in anal penetration, too, and never use anything without a substantially wider base than the anal opening (butt plugs and dildos have bases and these prevent objects disappearing up the rectum).

With anal sex and play, like any other aspects of sex, each partner must respect the boundaries set by the other and communication is as crucial as trust. Experimenting with penetration of any kind can be fun and allows each partner to have their sexual boundaries pushed a little. If your lover isn't comfortable with what's going on and doesn't want to continue, don't insist or try to coax her, just stop immediately.

Sex toys

While not all of us use sex toys, they do play a significant role in lesbian sex. We like toys because they widen the range of possible positions and sexual pleasures open to us; they can be used alone, or with company. The array of toys open to us is now huge, and instead of being things that were once bought surreptitiously, we can now buy them in high street stores. Some women might feel uncomfortable buying toys in a mixed store, but an increasing amount of women-only shops are opening to take account of this – check lesbian magazines or the Internet to find out where these shops are. People who work in reputable sex shops are there to help you. They won't get embarrassed by your questions and a good shop should be comfortable and the staff approachable and friendly. Magazines and the Internet are also useful for women who want to shop by mail order (now a blossoming industry). They are ideal for women who can't get to a shop or who might feel shy about visiting a sex shop. The packaging is very discreet, so no one will know what is being brought to your home.

Sex toys come in almost every imaginable size, shape, colour and material, which can make choosing them a bit confusing. It might help, beforehand, to work out what you want. Is it something you'll want to use alone, or would you like to share it with a lover? Do you both want to use it at the same time? How much do you want to pay? Try to imagine what uses you could put the toy to and get advice from the sales staff.

After use, clean all your toys carefully and don't use them straight from one woman to another – this will help prevent bacterial infections (such as yeast infections) being spread from woman to woman. Cleaning methods depend on what the toy is made of. When you buy your items, check with the shop or the manufacturer for any particular cleaning instructions. In general, though, silicone can be boiled (you can actually put it in the dishwasher for a few minutes) in order to sterilize it. Latex and rubber jelly or PVC toys, however, should only be washed in hot water with a very mild soap. Toys that have been in the anus or around the anal opening should never be used in or near the vagina and if you have one toy being shared between two partners, use a new condom on the toy before it is used by either woman.

BELOW Toys can bring a lot of added pleasure to sex and they allow for experimentation with new positions and sensations. These days, the range is so vast that just about everything you can imagine (and some things you won't have thought of) is available.

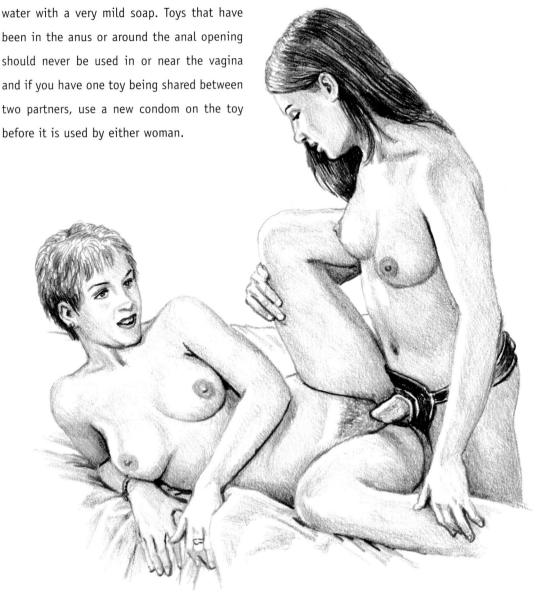

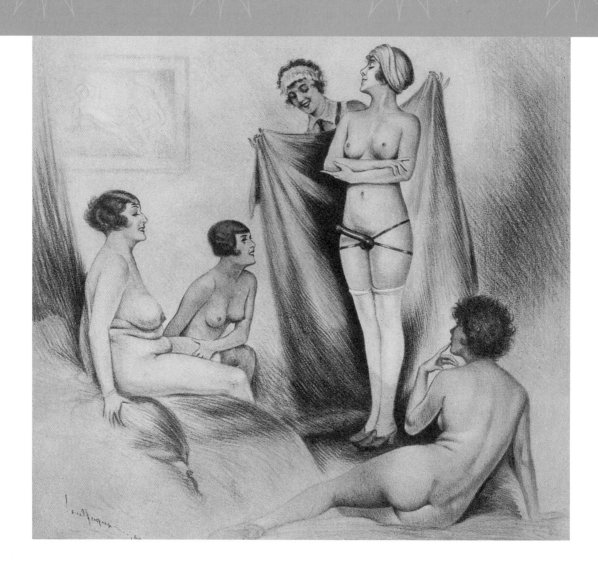

ABOVE 'Men, Who Needs Them?' by Eugène Reunier. Buying a sex toy can often be an intimidating or nerve-racking experience. Staff at reputable shops know this and will do all they can to make you feel at ease. Don't be embarrassed to ask questions or for advice. You are not the only person to enter a sex shop and yours won't be the first questions or concerns the staff have heard.

Dildos and vibrators

Vibrators are probably still the most popular sex toy, varying in power from quite vigorous to less intense. They can be placed directly on the clitoris and vulva, or inside you. Most are battery operated and many manufacturers now make waterproof versions that can be taken into the bath or shower. A particularly popular brand of vibrator is the 'Rabbit', so-named because, while it has the usual long shaft, it has an additional piece shaped like little rabbit ears to stimulate the clitoris. Vibrators are very versatile: some are pocket-sized; others can be fitted into a harness; the G-spot vibrator is curved at the end to enable deep penetration in the G-spot area; there are multi-speed vibrators, clit massagers and vibrators that can be attached to a finger.

Dildos, on the other hand, are solid and do not vibrate. They can be either hand-held or worn in harnesses and come in a variety of sizes and shapes; whereas most dildos were once made to resemble penises, they now come in a vast array of designs and textures. You can buy dildos for single penetration, curved for G-spot penetration, or ridged or shaped for extra stimulation. There are double-ended dildos – these tend to be very long because one end is intended to be inserted into one partner while the other end goes into the other woman. Double dildos are also available in a curved L-shape so that when fitted into a harness, one end can penetrate the harness wearer while the other is used to penetrate her partner.

Harnesses also come in a variety of styles, most being made from leather or a synthetic material. Apart from the traditional strap and buckles harness, you can also get thong harnesses, corset harnesses and strap-on-thigh harnesses, where the dildo is positioned on the front of the thigh (this is good for penetration when there's a height difference between women).

Plugs, clamps and restraining equipment

Toys for anal play include butt plugs, which come in a variety of shapes and sizes, and double-ended anal toys, (these require a good level of coordination with your lover). Anal wands are long, thin strips of plastic, ridged with rounded beads. If inserted into a partner's anus, an anal wand can give an overwhelming sensation when pulled out quickly. For the nipples there are clamps – adjustable, vibrating screw clamps and, for the more adventurous, weighted clamps (care should be taken not to damage the nipples when using clamps). Those into correction, or even just fun spanking, could consider whips and paddles. Whips will vary, but fetish shops tend to stock a much more hard-core selection. A paddle is a hand-held, oar-shaped piece of leather or plastic, which is used to spank. Again, fetish stores sell heavier-duty paddles. Cuffs and restraints can vary considerably in quality, so check them out before you buy. Some handcuffs might be padded for comfort while others are plain metal.

Piercings

In the lesbian and gay culture, piercing is a popular form of body adornment, along with tattooing. During the 1980s and early 1990s, body piercing was very common on the gay scene. Since then, it's become a mainstream fashion statement. While having your body pierced can be an extremely exhilarating thing to do, it's important that it's done correctly. Never pierce anything yourself. Unclean needles can pass on such diseases as Hepatitis B and C, HIV and other infections. Body piercing should be done by a reputable and certified practitioner. A good professional will give you all the advice you need and won't persuade you to go through with it, if you change your mind.

Quite a few lesbians choose to have their nipples pierced, and nipple jewellery comes in the form of a ring closed by a small metal ball or a metal barbell. Many women pierce their nipples because they believe it can make this part of the body more sensitive, especially when the piercing is being played with. While this can sometimes be true, piercing can also lessen the feeling in the nipple (however, it may then increase the sensitivity in the unpierced nipple). Some people want nipple rings to be decorative and don't care about the loss of sensitivity, but it's a good idea to have one nipple pierced at a time – that way, you won't risk losing sensitivity in both.

Over the past few years the number of women with genital piercing has grown. Most are performed through the clit hood or the clitoris itself, through the inner and outer labia, or through the base of the vaginal opening and perineum. Like nipple rings, piercings in this area can heighten arousal, physically and psychologically. Piercings look sexy, and can be erotic during sex – a nipple ring traced over the aroused clit of a lover, or used to rub her nipple, can be a huge turn on. But the jewellery must be kept clean. Wash a ring with warm water and a gentle soap if it's been on your lover's genitals, and avoid harsh, over-perfumed soaps. If it looks as though a piercing might be causing problems, such as infection, swelling or redness in the surrounding area, take it out or have a professional remove it.

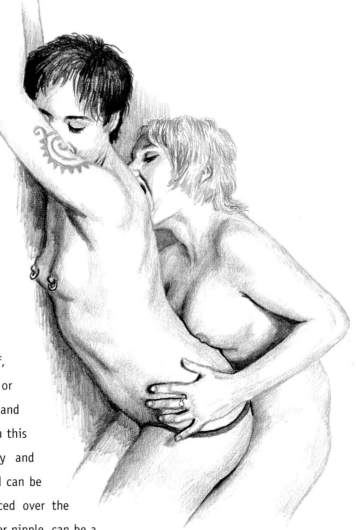

ABOVE Piercings – when done safely and cleanly – can add an interesting dimension to sex play and offer increased sensitivity to the nipples, clit hood or labia.

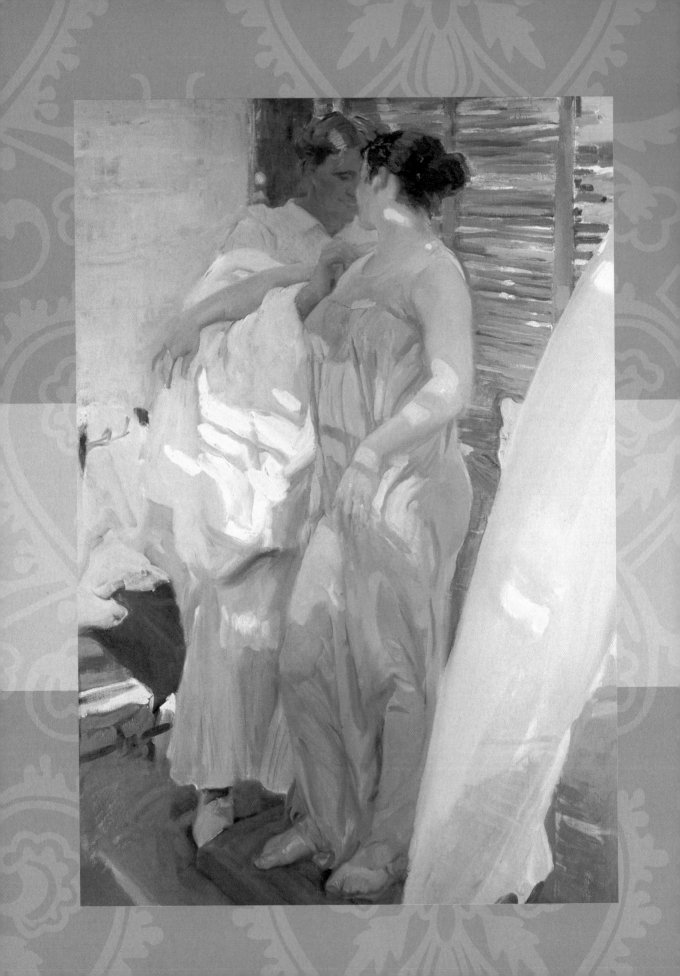

Chapter 5:
For women only:
The facts you need

coming out

coming out

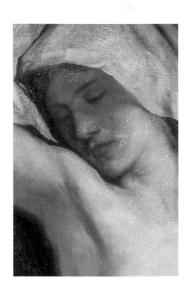

Admitting that you might be gay or that you find other women sexually attractive may be terrifying at first, and telling a friend or family member about your sexuality can seem intimidating, or even impossible.

ABOVE Coming out about your sexuality is probably one of the hardest things any lesbian has to do. And you don't just come out once; you come out day after day to all sorts of people in all walks of life. People who are not gay will never understand how difficult it can be and the effects it can have.

OPPOSITE 'Two Ladies on a Swing' from 'Les Sylphides' engraving by Charles Bargue (1826–83). Meeting other women for friendship or sex can be difficult, but these days there are many ways to do it, either in person through social groups, bars and clubs or through contact ads in lesbian magazines and on websites.

There are other aspects about 'coming out' that are equally daunting. Information about social activities, the difficulties you may face in a largely heterosexual world, your legal rights and healthcare geared specifically for you may be difficult to find. Dating women and exploring your sexuality while maintaining good sexual health will play an important part in your development and give you an opportunity to know yourself. Forming relationships, whether short- or long-term, will help to shape your life and give it meaning. Attending to your physical and mental health makes you a strong, self-assured and confident woman and contributes to your happiness throughout all the changing phases of your life.

Meeting other women

Okay, so you've come out, but where are your playmates? It's likely you'll want to meet new people, especially if you don't have any lesbian friends already, or you might want to meet someone for sex.

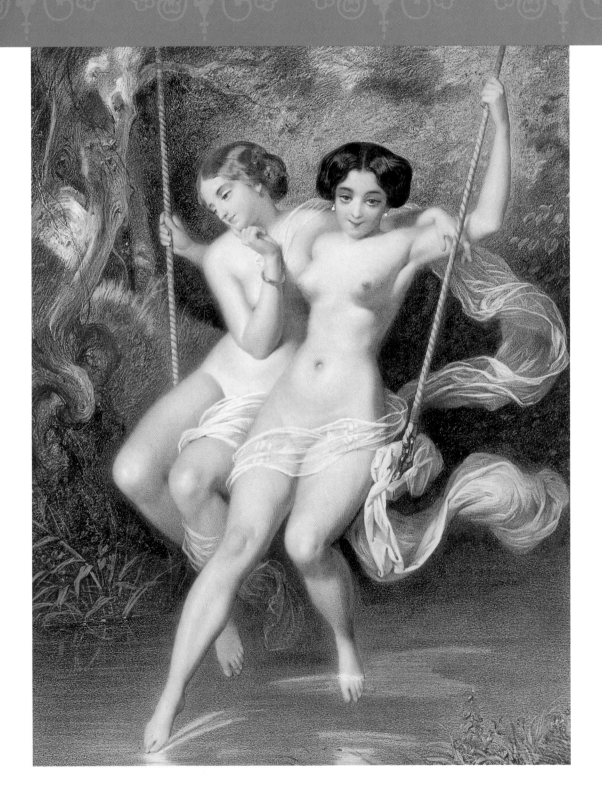

Later on, you may be interested in dating or finding a girlfriend. Obviously, it's going to be easier to meet women if you live in a city with a thriving lesbian and gay scene, but even if you live somewhere less populated and more isolated, it's easier than ever before to make contact with other women. Internet sites, lesbian magazines and city guides carry information on all sorts of social groups, not just bars and clubs. These organizations can be specifically aimed at people just coming out, or there are sports, leisure, social, debating, political and even religious groups, depending on your favourite pursuits. It's not hard to find a club for just about any interest or age range, and it's a good way to meet like-minded friends or develop a support network. Such organizations can also enable you to make friends if you've just moved to the area, or want to meet new people after a relationship break-up.

If nothing appeals to you locally, get online and talk to other women in the many chatrooms that exist. You might find other lesbians who live near you and maybe you could get together for a coffee or an evening out. If you become friendly with women who live further away, make the effort to schedule time together. Another option is to meet through personal ads, either placing your own or answering someone else's. Many mainstream magazines now have a 'Women seeking Women' column in their personals section and also carry listings of lesbian and gay bars, clubs and events.

Meeting new friends makes it easier to go out and find women for sex and dating because you've got someone to accompany you to bars or clubs. Going alone is hard and can be depressing because the lesbian scene, like any other, can sometimes be rather hostile and unfriendly to women on their own. Your friends will have other friends and they can introduce you to other women they may know.

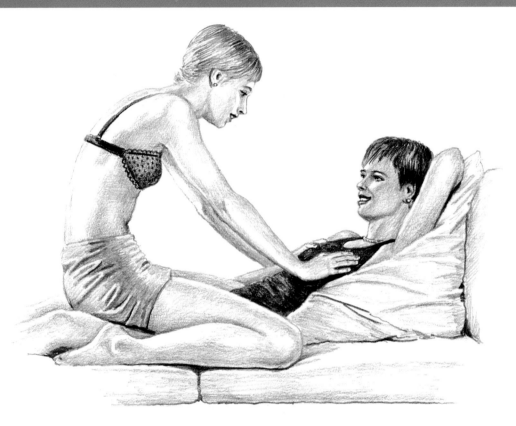

You might be able to meet women for sex and dating through social networks and groups, but bars play a big part in lesbian culture. They're good places to flirt, dance, enjoy yourself in the company of other women and, if you're lucky, meet someone for sex. If you live in a place where there's a busy, thriving lesbian scene, there will probably be bars that cater for different interests and tastes, such as dance clubs, bars for older women or those into S&M, venues that hold line-dancing nights and places that are more 'cruisey'. Some localities may only have one gay bar or even an occasional night at a regular club. Women's social nights at bars can also be a good way of meeting friends, rather than just scouting for sex. A word of caution: while alcohol is good for getting the conversation flowing and lowering your inhibitions, be

ABOVE Getting to know someone, both physically and emotionally, is important for a healthy sex life and relationship. Sometimes lovers are right for us, sometimes they are not, and we all make mistakes on that journey of discovery.

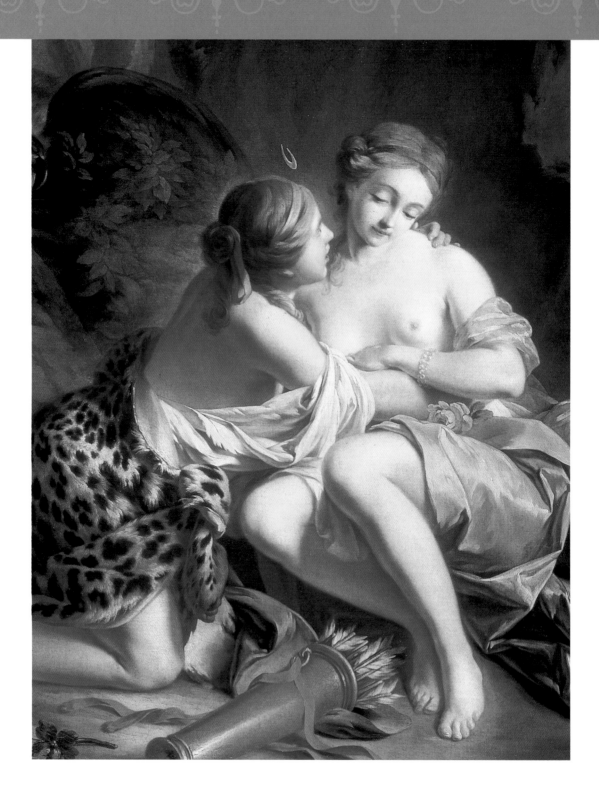

careful that you don't get too carried away. Nervousness can make you drink more, so try to keep it within safe limits to avoid endangering yourself when it comes to taking chances with whom you leave and how you get home.

Teen sex

The first real interest in sex normally begins with puberty and coincides with the development of sexual identity. For the lesbian teen, becoming aware of her sexuality, let alone 'coming out', can be difficult, and no teen wants to stand out from her peers. However, with more lesbian and gay youth groups, improved sex education and the increased representation of lesbians in the media, teenagers can feel more confident about coming out. Currently, most countries don't have a specific age of consent on lesbian sex; legislators in the past might have thought it didn't go on.

While some girls can cope with their sexual identity, others say they are bisexual, fearing less peer disapproval. But teenage sex brings with it a whole host of emotions because it's so new. You've met someone and they want to have sex with you: ask yourself if you are ready. Don't be pressured into it by someone else, but only do what makes you feel comfortable. Making love when both partners are uneasy could make the experience less than wonderful, which might make you feel bad. Accept that you could be nervous, and so could the other girl, especially if it's your first time. Sometimes the initial encounter can be a bit disappointing, but try again and learn to laugh about any silly misadventures that might arise. Treat a lover as you'd like to be treated. Make sure you trust her and be aware that you have the right to stop if you change your mind. This is the beginning of your life-long sexual adventure.

OPPOSITE 'Jupiter and Callisto' by Jean-Simon Berthelemey (1743–1811). Our first sexual encounter might not be the best sex of our lives, but it is among the most important. We can be at our most emotionally vulnerable when young – our bodies, sexual urges and thoughts are so new that they can seem overwhelming.

BELOW The original Kama Sutra firmly believes that a relationship should enrich us, not just sexually, but also emotionally. A fulfilling partnership can sometimes be difficult to find, and equally hard to maintain. It requires time, patience and respect.

Relationships

Almost all of us have had a relationship at some point. Monogamous or 'open', they can last a lifetime or just a few weeks. Whatever the relationship you share with another women, each partner should aim not only to pleasure the other's body, but also to enhance and enrich each other's mind and spirits. The fundamental message at the heart of the Kama Sutra is not one of selfish love, but rather all-encompassing love. It should involve passion of the body and mind equally, and not just for the individual – good sex is about sharing an emotion and an experience with someone else, not just deriving quick pleasure for yourself. It is also about respect. Whether short- or long-term, the women involved should treat each other and the relationship with respect.

Some women happen to be fortunate enough to find the right partner early on, others flit from one lover to the next, searching for the right person, while still more leave one relationship only to enter into another one immediately afterwards. Relationships work and fail for many different reasons. Be prepared to acknowledge that your lover might not be prepared to commit to anyone, ever, or maybe just not to you. It's a wonderful and fulfilling feeling when a relationship works out but it can sometimes feel like the worst experience in the world when it fails or ends. This applies especially if it's your first relationship, one in which you've been for a long time, or if you've been building up your hopes about someone without being entirely realistic.

For various reasons, certain relationships succeed and are happy, just as others are unhappy and may end. When a relationship finishes, it can be devastating, but try not to beat yourself up about it, or feel like a failure. The relationship might not have been right for you or healthy; you may have tried to connect to the other person and not succeeded. The other woman might have let you down, or maybe you let them down. Perhaps you can part on good terms, even though you don't intend to see each other again, but sometimes the hurt which is left doesn't make that possible.

Keeping passion alive

The beginning of a relationship can be the most exciting part: the anticipation of meeting for dates, the mutual passion and sex that is fast, furious and delicious. The passion may be easy to keep up in the early stages, but like all relationships that extend over a period of time, things change and evolve. Partners don't always move from one phase to another at the same time, which can lead to misunderstandings. One partner might still want lots of urgent, passionate sex, while the other has moved beyond that to a greater emotional involvement.

Problems may also arise when one partner has a higher sex drive and wants sex more often. If the other woman rejects her lover's advances, this may result in feelings of confusion and hurt. Feeling guilty or a sense that she feels you're letting her down may lead you to having sex with your lover when you really don't want to. While this may work occasionally, long-term it will damage your self-esteem and relationship. If you want less or more sex than your lover, there's nothing wrong with you – you just need to explain how you feel. Gently tell your lover that you are still attracted to her, but that you don't share the same levels of sexual desire. If the relationship is to succeed, communication is crucial. You each need to be honest about what you want and expect emotionally and sexually from the relationship, and from each other.

A loss of sexual passion is often the first thing to suffer in a long-term relationship – it even has the name 'lesbian bed death' – so keeping sex exciting or even regular can be challenging. Over long periods of time, the responsibilities of daily life – work, finances and children, to name but a few – can get in the way of sex. There are ways around this, but they require imagination from both partners. Try to make time for each other away from the stresses and distractions of the day. Go out for a leisurely dinner and flirt with each other; act like it's your first date and you're just getting to know her – you might remind yourself of the reason you fell for her in the first place. Consider signing up for a course together on a common interest that will involve close interaction, such as taking a foreign language or dancing class. Or learn how to perform sensual massage and set aside a few hours once a week to practise on each other. You could buy a new sex toy together and go away for the weekend to try it out, read erotica out loud to each other, pretend you're strangers and meet for a date and illicit sex, or simply watch a lesbian porn film together. Take inspiration from the Kama Sutra, which encourages the study of arts and sciences in order to develop into a well-rounded and versatile lover. Known as the 64 arts, these include such activities as singing, dancing, playing a musical instrument, writing and drawing, cooking, decorating, gardening, languages and sports, as well as more esoteric subjects.

Another way to rediscover your sexual side comes in the form of Tantric sex, the ancient philosophy that aims to unite two lovers through energy. Tantra has less to do with the genitals and orgasms and more with uniting the body and mind in a spiritually fulfilling experience. The discipline centres around food and sex rituals, concentrating on the cleansing of the body and consciously introducing or eradicating certain foods from your diet as well as focusing on the sensual aspects of lovemaking. It's a good way for lovers who have become distant to reconnect and use their mutual sexual energy in a totally different way. A number of health, wellbeing and spirituality centres now organize courses on practising this art. Tantra directly relates to one of the main précis of the Kama

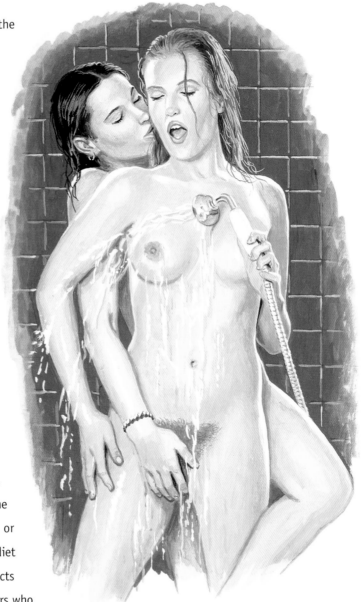

ABOVE Trying new sensations and more unusual locations for lovemaking will help to keep the passion alive in a relationship.

Sutra: the enjoyment of the object, in this case, the lover, by the five senses of hearing, feeling, seeing, tasting, and smelling, assisted by the mind, together with the soul.

However you reconnect with your lover, the key is to make time for each other away from normal routines, to try and understand each other's needs and to make an effort. A good relationship should allow each person to grow and become fulfilled as an independent individual rather than just part of the unit. If, despite making an effort, difficulties persist, then there might be deeper, more underlying problems in your relationship. Sorting through them yourself may be difficult, and seeking professional help could be a workable option. There's no shame in couples counselling – having an independent person talk through your problems with you might help get your relationship back on track again.

Sex and menstruation

Having sex during your monthly cycle may make you self-conscious about the blood or smell, or worried about staining the sheets. This, again, is a time for communication between lovers. Does your lover want you to go down on her while she's menstruating? Do you like being penetrated while bleeding, or does your vagina become sore? There's no reason not to have oral sex during a period unless there's a risk that one partner may pass on a sexually transmitted infection/disease (STI/STD) to the other, as menstrual blood is an effective bodily fluid for transmission.

Talk and find out what you both like. It's not uncommon to find that your sex drive increases considerably just before you get a period. This can continue during menstruation, or you may find that sexual desire is lost amid all the cramps. There's a commonly held belief that orgasms are good for getting rid of period cramps, though some women would swear it only makes them worse. When two women live together, it's not uncommon for them to find that their periods synchronize, which is good news if you both get increased sex drives before menstruating, but a nightmare if you suffer from Pre-Menstrual Syndrome/Tension (PMS/PMT).

Sex and pregnancy

Over the last few years, lesbian mothers have become more visible in the media and in ordinary day-to-day life. With increased rights and access to fertility services, more lesbians are deciding to have children, with a partner or as a single parent. Women may choose to co-parent with a gay male friend who donates the sperm (usually for self-insemination), or the mother might use an anonymous sperm donor through a fertility clinic because she does not want contact with the biological father. It is also not uncommon now to see both the women in a relationship give birth to children. Increasing numbers of lesbians are choosing to become mothers, so sex during pregnancy is an issue that will get more exposure in lesbian publications.

There are huge hormonal and physical changes in a woman's body during the first three months of pregnancy. This is the time when the oestrogen and progesterone levels rocket and women may find their sex drives plummet or soar because of the extra oestrogen. Breasts get considerably larger and, by the second trimester, there are increased blood flows to the vulva, engorging the erectile tissue. This can allow for new types of sexual stimulation, which some women say results in greater arousal and stronger orgasms. The additional oestrogen also increases vaginal lubrication.

A foetus is well protected by the uterus, and so there's no chance that it can be harmed by orgasms or penetration, even into the third trimester. The bigger the woman's bump gets, the more comfort plays a part in sexual positions. Some activities, such as fisting, should not be tried during pregnancy or for some time after birth. Sex during and after pregnancy, is the subject of specialist books, and further reading is recommended (see also page 144).

Sex and the menopause

The transition from being reproductive to non-reproductive happens when the ovaries stop producing oestrogen and progesterone. A woman will usually start to display pre-menopausal symptoms around three or five years before her last period. The menopause can occur any time between the mid-40s and the late 50s, but it's not uncommon for it to occur much earlier in some women. Certain illnesses or cancer treatments may affect the menopause, as does the removal of the ovaries, or a hysterectomy. It also appears earlier in women who smoke.

Because of the decrease of oestrogen and progesterone, women may find their sexual desires diminish. Among hot flushes, depression, mood swings, becoming hairier and an end to periods, other drawbacks of the menopause include the reduction in vaginal lubrication and the thinning of the vaginal canal, which can both make penetration painful. These days, however, there are a number of very good artificial lubricants to use during sex that can now be bought in pharmacies and they will make sex feel less uncomfortable. If you use sex toys, you will find that a smaller one is more comfortable as the menopause approaches. Because of the thinning of the vaginal walls, fisting and vigorous sex become more difficult.

The menopause is not known as 'The Change' without good reason. Not only does a woman's body go through huge physical changes, but there will also be psychological changes to take into account. What you like sexually may alter, as may your libido and the frequency with which you want sex. The feelings you have about the ageing of your body shouldn't be underestimated, either. For some women, this can be a difficult time, and if this applies to you, don't shut your lover out. This can often be challenging for the partner who is not experiencing the menopause, too, especially if there's an age gap in a relationship. Accept that there will be changes, and don't spend too much time mourning about how you used to feel; instead, concentrate your energy on learning new sexual responses.

Bisexuality

This is a curious subject in the lesbian and gay world. Bisexuality can meet with a great deal of disapproval, particularly in some sections of the lesbian community. There's a lot of stereotyping of bisexual women – that they're untrustworthy and less reliable, that they want the 'best of both worlds', that they'll leave you for a man, that they're sexually promiscuous, and so on. Of course these are all myths and, like lesbians or straight women, bisexual women are all different. There's no hard and fast rule about what a bisexual is and how they behave, any more than there is about how lesbians should act.

For many women, especially during adolescence, bisexuality may act as a transition phase: the bridge between 'heterosexuality' and being lesbian or gay. Others remain bisexual – that is, either sexually attracted to or sexually active with both sexes – throughout their lives. In the past five or six years, the bisexual community has really begun to emerge, and there are movements

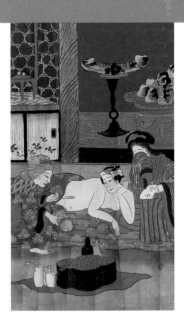

ABOVE A detail from 'The Island of Women', *c* 1870. Shunga prints like this one were often bound together in book form and sold as sexual education manuals as well as explicit erotic art.

BELOW S&M can be fulfilling for many women, and the bondage gear may add a sense of fun and danger. But make sure that you trust your partner and are confident she knows what she's doing.

and organizations offering specific support and social networks. A greater tolerance is growing towards bisexuality and younger women tend to take it in their stride. If you feel you might be bisexual, try to find a support group geared to understanding what you're going through. At this stage, finding a lesbian group might not be quite what you need. Check online for your nearest group or any bisexual resource services. Many mainstream and lesbian publications carry contact/personal ads for bisexual women and support organizations. If you are having sex with men as well as women, you should make sure that you're taking relevant precautions when it comes to safer sex (see pages 133–5).

Sadomasochism

Commonly known as S&M, sadomasochism can take many forms. It may be something as simple as handcuffing your lover during sex, or as forceful as whipping or flagellating. It can involve engaging in extreme 'torture' play involving masks, chains and implements. The sadist is the one inflicting the pain; the masochist, the one who submits to, or receives it. Some of the very basic principles of kinky play appeal to a large number of people and even the mildest of sexual activities can contain elements of restraint and coercion – pinning a lover down, biting, scratching and spanking, for example – many of which are detailed in the Kama Sutra. Some people like to take S&M a stage further and move from bondage and restraints

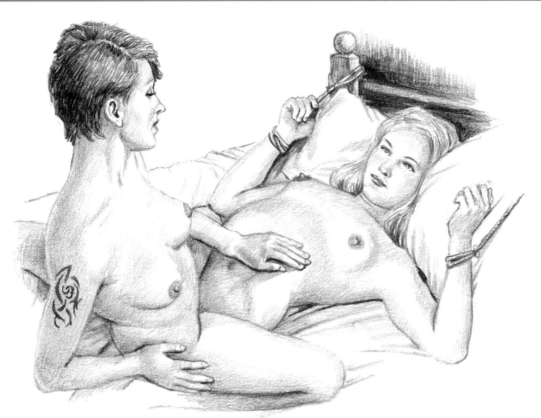

(ropes, chains and handcuffs), on to sensory deprivation (masks, gags and hoods) or more hardcore equipment.

Trust is a crucial aspect of S&M activity. Before either partner engages in any form of S&M play, negotiation must take place between couples. How far does each partner want to go? What do they expect to get out of it? Who's inflicting the pain? While one partner might consent to what's going on, there needs to be a 'stop' – or safe – word that will end the play immediately when their pain or sensory threshold is reached. This word is agreed before the play begins and once it is used, the activity must end immediately. Words with a sexual connotation or 'yes' or 'no' are unacceptable. Instead, partners agree a term among themselves using innocuous, often meaningless, words such as 'apple'.

ABOVE The use of restraints during sex can give you both an erotic charge, but you need mutual trust and consent. When one partner has had enough, the other must release her immediately. Keep scissors handy in case a restraint becomes too tight and cannot be unknotted.

Submission and domination (called Sub/Dom) play, where the dominant partner exercises control over the other, can often incorporate humiliation and the use of restraints in sex. It can be a huge turn-on for the women involved. Other women, however, become very excited by the idea of bondage. Tying up your lover, or being tied up while they tease you, can feel very sexy. Materials such as leather, silk and even metal offer different sensations and levels of pleasure against the skin. Blindfolds can add an additional excitement, because the wearer doesn't know what to expect next. If you are restraining a lover, make sure that the binding is not too tight as it can restrict or stop circulation. Be sure that you have some way of cutting the restraints, if an emergency should arise. Experimentation with sexual play allows both partners to discover what they like and their limitations. It can also be exciting to switch your traditional roles as a couple. Once you get used to being open with your lover in this way, you will almost certainly find it easier to say what you want in the relationship as a whole.

Games of power and restraint, like S&M, work on the same principles of trust and consent. They can also involve humiliation rather than actual physical pain, as in master/slave scenarios. In all cases, avoid getting involved with someone you don't know well or don't trust – you need to know the person will stop when you've had enough. It goes without saying that you should avoid drugs and drink when engaging in S&M. Both can numb the pain receptors and lower your awareness of how much pain is being inflicted. You might also agree to something you'd normally never consider. If you suspect the person dominating you or inflicting pain isn't sure what they're doing, get them to stop at once. Never let a partner pressure you into something you don't want to do.

Threesomes

You and two gorgeous women, all of you naked and getting up to all kinds of fun together, sounds like the stuff that fantasies are made of. Yes, threesomes can be an enjoyable and liberating experience, but there are some considerations you should take into account before you engage in one. Are you going to involve your lover and a third party, or do you want a threesome with two unattached women? Are you planning to make it a regular occurrence, should you find the right people, or is it to be a one-time-only event? While it might seem like a good idea to have a threesome with a partner, this can lead to jealousy issues. In theory, you might think you are fine about seeing someone going down on your lover, kissing her or penetrating her with a dildo, but in reality you may feel differently. Even if the three of you don't know each other well, jealousy can still arise. What if one woman is giving the other more attention than she's giving you? And what happens if they're really attracted to each other, and you feel like a spare part? If you discuss the idea first and prepare yourself for these eventualities, then threesomes can be a wonderful opportunity for experimentation and imagination. You might not feel jealous at all, and be far more worried about the delightful 'problem' of how to penetrate two women at the same time or keep up a constant rhythm!

BELOW Threesomes can be a fantastic experience, but they can be complicated, too, particularly if they involve your long-term partner. If the threesome is a spontaneous and uncomplicated act, then enjoy it! Relaxation and honesty play important roles, and an open mind and sense of adventure are a bonus.

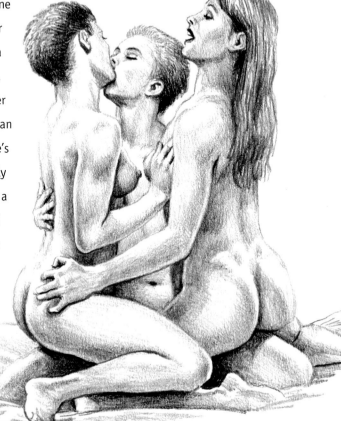

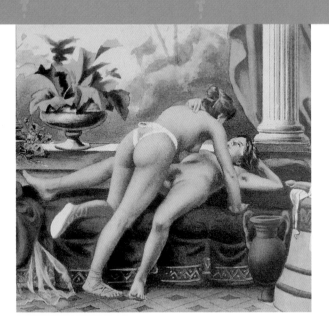

ABOVE 'Ancient Times' from the nineteenth-century *De Figuris Veneris* (A Manual of Classic Erotology) by Friedrich Karl Forberg. Just because we don't sleep with men, it doesn't mean we are not susceptible to certain sexually transmitted infections. Our bodies are our own responsibility and practising 'safer' sex will help protect against possible risks.

General healthcare

The Kama Sutra is a manual concerned with all aspects of love and the sexual experience. Not only does it promote an open, healthy attitude towards your sexual impulses, but it also urges individuals to attend to their mental and physical needs. Many aspects of healthcare are the same for straight and lesbian women. Make sure you have a regular Pap test, also known as a cervical smear test. Every two years is usual for women aged between 20 and 65, but recommendations vary according to the country in which you reside. Some people erroneously believe that lesbians are less at risk of cervical cancer because they don't sleep with men, and if you find your doctor is unhappy to perform regular tests, find another doctor or clinic.

Every woman should examine her own breasts regularly. It's important to realize how your breasts look and feel normally, so you are aware of any changes. While survival rates for breast cancer are higher than they've ever been before, there's a lot to be said for the power of prevention over cure. Avoid checking your breasts during a period, as some women experience swelling of the breasts. Stand in front of a mirror, lift up your arms and study your breasts and the armpit area from different angles. Look for lumps, bumps, any skin colouring changes or puckering. Check your nipples, too, for discharge or any skin or colour change. Most breast lumps, when tested, turn out to be benign (non-cancerous), but if you do find one, don't delay in seeking medical advice.

Safer sex

During the 1980s and early 1990s, healthcare agencies and the gay press talked about 'safe' sex. Over the past few years, the emphasis has shifted increasingly towards 'safer' sex. We now accept there's no such thing as 'safe' when it comes to sex with another person. Regardless of your sexuality or sexual preferences, there's always some risk of transmitting infections – it's the nature of human contact.

Each one of us has our unique personal history; many lesbians have slept with men in the past, and some will continue to do so. Other women might be bisexual and sleep regularly with both sexes. Only celibacy can offer 100 per cent safety and the next best thing is long-term monogamy with a partner whom you know is uninfected (although there are still infections you can pass to each other). If you have a lot of partners or are taking risks, get annual tests for sexually transmitted infections (STIs), also called sexually transmitted diseases (STDs) (see pages 136–40).

Communication

You have a moral responsibility to inform a sexual partner if you have any STIs so that you both can take the appropriate precautions to help minimize any risk of passing on an infection to the other person. However, if someone hasn't told you, never assume they're not infected. It's a sad fact of life, but people aren't always honest about their status. And just because you think you know someone and have built up a relationship with them, this doesn't mean you have to take risks with your safety. Alcohol and drugs can also impair your judgement when it comes to safer sex and it's worth bearing in mind that you might take risks when you are under the influence that you'd never normally consider.

BELOW Taking responsibility for our own sexual health and safety means that we should tell a partner if we have any infections we can pass on to them. If you have a long-standing or recurring problem, it is better to tell a new lover before you get too physically involved.

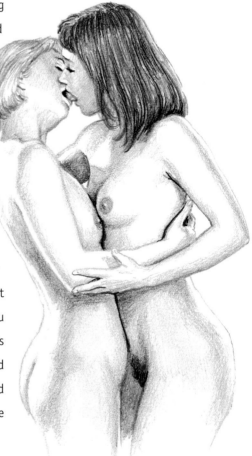

Methods of protection

There are a few precautions women should take to afford safety and protection when they have sex with another woman. Use your common sense to protect yourself and your partner from infection. Blood and vaginal secretions can harbour all major kinds of sexual or bacterial infections, which can be passed on to a sexual partner. Therefore, good sense should tell you that having broken or cut skin can be a perfect way for bacteria and infection to be transmitted, and this applies to your hands, mouth (including cracked lips), vagina or anus. There are ways to minimize risk. These include not sharing or mingling bodily fluids, not sharing sex toys that are unprotected or unclean, not touching someone's vagina or anus directly if you have cuts on the hand or fingers, and not having unprotected oral sex. The last of these applies especially during menstruation if the partner performing the sex act has cuts, gum disease or ulcers in the mouth.

Similarly, if you have a cold sore, don't go down on a partner or perform anilingus (rimming) on her, even with a dental dam because genital/anal and oral herpes are two different strains and an oral virus can change. If you have a cold sore (oral herpes), don't kiss your partner or touch your own mouth with your fingers, then finger your vagina or anus. If you're not using dental dams, don't go down on someone if you have a yeast infection in your mouth, or perform anilingus if the area is not clean enough.

Dental dams

These can be used during oral sex or anilingus. They are squares of latex (used by dentists during dental treatments, hence the name), which can be placed over the clitoris, vulva or anus to act as a barrier to bodily fluids. You can buy them from women's sex shops and they're sometimes available from sexual health clinics. If you can't find any, a spermicide-free condom cut down the middle works just as well. Most women would agree that dental dams are pretty dreadful; they're rather thick and often don't taste very nice, but until something better is invented for use among women for safer sex, they offer a good form of protection from fluids and infections.

Condoms

Apart from their use as makeshift dental dams, condoms play another crucial role in woman-to-woman safer sex. They should always be used on dildos or vibrators if they are being shared between partners, and change condoms if you switch from using a toy in your vagina to your anus. Any woman who still has sex with men must use a condom to protect themselves, as the risks of contracting an infection are higher between men and women.

Gloves

There's something very sexy about a well-lubed latex glove – the smoothness can feel wonderful for the woman being touched or penetrated. Gloves are easy to buy and you can get them in pharmacies. Make sure your nails aren't too long because this can tear the fingertips, especially while engaged in thrusting your finger inside a lover. Gloves are highly recommended for vaginal fisting, as the latex makes the hand smoother and therefore easier to get inside (always use lots of lube when engaging in fisting). Change gloves if you are transferring from vaginal to anal sex. If you are sharing a butt plug during anal play, wrap a plug in one of the glove's fingers and then wrap the rest of the glove around the base.

Sexually transmitted infections

As a lesbian, you may have found yourself in the frustrating situation in which medical professionals have assumed that, because you don't have sex with men, you are at less risk of contracting a sexually transmitted infection (STI). In the past, organizations promoting safer-sex awareness tended to overlook woman-to-woman transmission of infections, especially in the UK, although the US has always had a more proactive stance on woman-to-woman safer sex. But lesbian sexual activity transmits infection just like everyone else, though the risk through all-female sex is not as great as in gay or heterosexual sex.

Lesbians can pass on some infections and diseases more easily than others. Contrary to what people think, lesbians can transmit HIV to each other, although we're considered a very low-risk group. Generally, statistics for such infections have been based on two factors: having sex with men and the use of intravenous drugs. However, HIV has been discovered in vaginal secretions and

BELOW While some infections are harder to transfer between women, others are only too easy. If you notice any unusual symptoms, the most common being discharge, itching or soreness, contact a doctor or sexual health clinic immediately. Most infections can be easily treated if you don't delay.

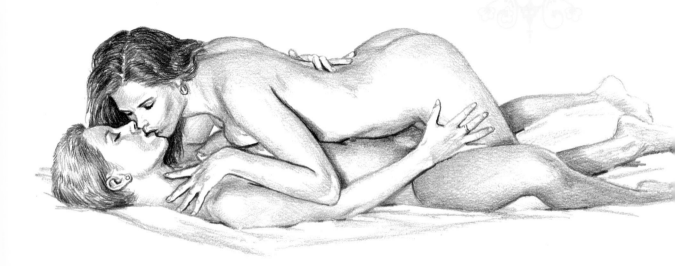

menstrual blood, and therefore sexual contact can provide a risk of transmission. Penetrating someone with a dildo/vibrator which has infected blood or vaginal fluid on it, or having unprotected oral sex/finger penetration during a period with a partner who has cuts in the mouth or on the hands are particular methods of infection.

Symptoms and treatments

Often STIs can have no single, obvious infection site, but if you experience itching, redness, an inflamed vulva, an unpleasant discharge or a nasty smell, chances are something is far from right. Don't feel embarrassed or ashamed if you contract an STI; there's nothing to feel bad about. Seek medical advice as soon as you notice a symptom. Leaving it will not make it go away, and will probably make it worse. Remember, gynaecologists, nurses and the professionals who work in sexual health clinics are used to seeing these types of problems, even if it's new to you. If you don't feel confident about visiting your doctor or gynaecologist, go to your nearest sexual health clinic where you can often be treated anonymously (see also page 144).

Chlamydia

Although the most common and most easily treated of STIs, chlamydia can be hard to detect because there are very few symptoms. Left untreated, it can lead to pelvic inflammation and, eventually, infertility. Symptoms (if any) include vaginal discharge, pain in the abdomen, bleeding or pain during penetrative sex or frequent and uncomfortable urinating. Chlamydia can be treated with antibiotics. Women who have unprotected sex with men should consider being tested for this condition.

Crabs

Pubic lice are tiny parasites that live mostly in the pubic hair, although they can spread to body hair. Look closely and you'll see little brown eggs on the hair and the lice themselves. They are usually passed on through contact during sex. Symptoms include itching and flaky skin. Treatment comes in the form of a non-prescription medicated lotion available from a pharmacist. Avoid sex for a week after completion of the treatment. Wash underwear, clothing, bedding and towels thoroughly in hot water.

Hepatitis

There are three types of the hepatitis virus: A, B and C, although A and B are of most consequence during sex. Hepatitis A is the most common type, the easiest to treat and the recovery rate is very high. It's transmitted through oral and anal contact – usually faecal matter – so could be passed through anilingus. It can also be passed on through contaminated food, such as uncooked shellfish, and water. Symptoms include fever, jaundice (a yellowing of the skin), tiredness, rashes, weight loss and fever. Infected individuals can infect others two weeks before feeling ill themselves.

Like hepatitis A, hepatitis B is discovered through a blood test. Hepatitis B is far more serious and is passed on in a similar way to HIV: through blood and bodily fluids. It can cause serious liver damage. Many people show no symptoms, but those who do display jaundice and a yellowing of the eyes, dark urine, pale stools, fever, rashes, aching, sickness and a flu-like state, which passes after a few weeks. Hepatitis B is more infectious than HIV and can be passed on through saliva, so even kissing and sharing a toothbrush or drink could transmit it from one partner to another.

If you think you may be at risk, or are planning travel to certain countries, ask your doctor about a vaccine. A low-fat diet and the avoidance of alcohol are recommended, as is lots of rest and medication under a doctor's guidance.

Herpes

After an initial outbreak, the herpes simplex virus lies dormant in the body. The sufferer may never experience another episode, but usually further outbreaks occur when the individual is run down, tired or depressed. Herpes is passed on through skin contact from the mouth, vagina or anus. There are two types: Type 1, which affects the mouth and the area around the nose, and is known as a cold sore, and Type 2, which appears

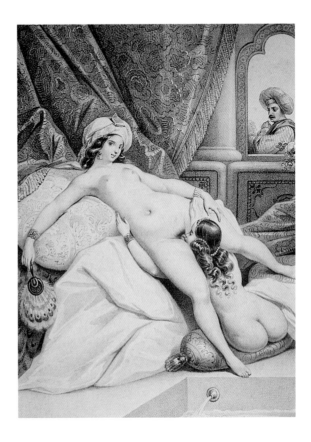

around the genital and anal areas. An outbreak is characterized by an itching or tingling sensation, followed by the appearance of small, fluid-filled blisters. These become highly infectious sores, before drying out into scabs. Genital herpes sufferers can also experience flu-like symptoms, swelling of the glands, headaches or fevers. If you get an outbreak, see a doctor for medication. You may find it recurs and, if so, it might require continual treatment.

ABOVE 'The Harem', an erotic lithograph by Achille Devéria (1800–1857). The pleasures of cunnilingus, like sex in general, carry physical risks. Knowledge is the key to protecting yourself and spotting any potential problems.

Genital warts

Caused by the human papilloma virus, genital warts appear as either small, pink-white lumps or larger, bumpy ones and are passed by hand-to-genital contact, skin-to-skin or hand-to-anal contact (warts can appear on the anus). They don't hurt but they do itch, and should be treated with antibiotics. If left untreated, the warts can become cancerous.

Gonorrhoea

Although rare in lesbians, any woman having sex with men should get herself tested for this particular bacterial infection. You may have no symptoms at all, but common ones include a yellowish discharge and painful urination. It is contagious, even if there are no symptoms. Treatment is by antibiotics.

Syphilis

This bacterial infection is now at epidemic levels in some parts of the UK and US. It's predominately passed through gay and straight sex, rather than lesbian sex. Untreated, syphilis may be deadly, although the initial symptoms can be few. Preliminary small, ulcerous growths on the vulva and anus are followed by secondary symptoms, which include a rash covering the body, flu-like illness, tiredness and swollen glands. It's highly contagious during the first stages, but can be treated with penicillin. If you think you may be at risk, and especially if you sleep with men, get tested regularly.

Trichomonas vaginalis

After infection, a sufferer may notice an unpleasant, greenish vaginal discharge and a strong smell. There can also be soreness around the vagina, itching and pain during sex and urination. Trichomonas vaginalis, called TV, is transmitted via sex, but also through sharing towels and washcloths. The treatment is with antibiotics.

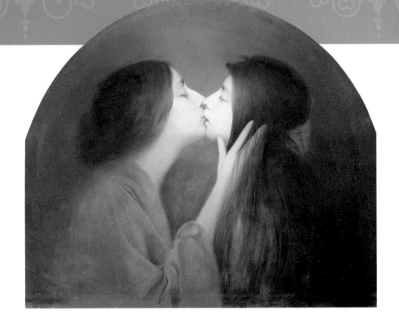

LEFT 'The Kiss' by Joseph Granie (1866–1915), *c* 1900. From the outset the Kama Sutra encouraged the world to view sex with joy and wonder, and to respect ourselves and those with whom we have sexual and emotional relationships. Two millennia on and this ethos is equally as important now as it was then.

The pursuit of happiness

Of course being a lesbian isn't just about sex, although it is, as we all know, an important part of life. We are all unique people, with our own particular combination of interests, needs and desires. The hope behind this book is to show how it's possible to integrate our sexual identity with other important aspects of our make-up, including health, self-esteem, emotions and relationships with other women. Being a well-rounded, centred individual is the basic, fundamental principle of the Kama Sutra and it still has as much relevance in this regard today as it did over 2,000 years ago. Only when we live full and contented lives do we have a chance of finding real happiness.

You can't type what what a lesbian is.
We're anything and everything.
The one thing in common is that we make love to other women.
So give up trying to limit us.

AMANDA BEARSE, ACTOR AND TELEVISION DIRECTOR

index

resources and acknowledgements

Further reading

Becoming Orgasmic, Julia R Heiman and Joseph LoPiccolo, Piatkus Books, 1988. Information on helping women to grow sexually.

Big O, The, Lou Paget, Piatkus Books, 2002. Everything you want to know about orgasms.

Bottoming Book, The, Dossie Easton and Catherine A Liszt, Greenery Press, 1995.

Change: Women, Ageing and the Menopause, The, Germain Greer, Ballantine Books, 1993.

Clitoral Truth, The, Rebecca Chalker, Seven Stories Press, 2002. A guide to the clitoris.

Come Hither: A Commonsense Guide to Kinky Sex, Dr Gloria G Brame, Fireside, 2000. From bondage and spanking to cross dressing – a guide for the curious.

Gay and Lesbian Online (fifth edition), Jeff Dawson, Alyson Publications, 2003. More than 4,000 gay and lesbian websites across the world, catering for every possible desire or need.

Good Vibrations Guide To Sex, The, Cathy Wink and Ann Semans, Cleis Press (third edition), 2002. One of the world's most popular sex manuals, which covers a huge number of subjects. www.cleispress.com

G-Spot, The, Alice Kahn Ladas, Beverly Whipple amd John D Perry, Henry Holt & Co, 1982. A guide on how to find your G-spot and stimulate it.

Joy of Lesbian Sex, The, Emily Sisley and Bertha Harris, Simon & Schuster, 1986.

Kama Sutra of Vatsyayana, The, Sir Richard Burton and FF Arbuthnot, Thorsons, 1997.

Lesbian Health Book The, Eds. Jocelyn White and Marissa C Martinez, Seal Press, 1997. An essential guide to lesbian health brought together by doctors, health workers and lesbians.

Lesbian Sex Book, The, Wendy Caster, Alyson Publications (second edition), 2003. A guide to all aspects of lesbian sex and intimacy. www.Alyson.com

Lesbian Sex, JoAnne Gardner Loulan, Spinster Book Company, 1985. Written by lesbians for lesbians.

A Mother's Guide to Sex, A, Anne Semans and Cathy Wink, Three Rivers Press, 2001. A guide to sex throughout motherhood.

New Topping Book, The, Dossie Easton and Catherine A Liszt, Greenery Press, 2001. A guide to S&M.

Pictures and Passions: A History of Homosexuality in the Visual Arts, James M Saslow, Viking, 1999.

Renaissance of Lesbianism in Early Modern England, The, Valerie Traub, Cambridge University Press, 2002.

Sex Book, The, Suzi Godson (with Mel Agace), Cassell Illustrated, 2003. A vastly comprensive guide to sex, sexuality, sexual health and emotions.

Sex for One, Betty Dodson, Random House Value Publications, 1996. One of the world's most famous sex experts gives advice on the joys of self-loving.

SM 101 – A Realistic Introduction, Jay Wiseman, Greenery Press, 1998.

Tickle Your Fancy: A Woman's Guide to Sexual Self Pleasure, Sadie Allison, Tickle Kitty Press, 2001.

Ultimate Guide to Anal Sex for Women, The, Tristan Taormino, Cleis Press, 1997.

Ultimate Guide to Cunnilingus, The, Violet Blue, Cleis Press, 2002. A guide on giving the best oral sex.

Ultimate Guide to Strap-On Sex, The, Karlyn Lotney, Cleis Press, 2000. A guide to dildos and harnesses.

Whole Lesbian Sex Book, The, Felice Newman, Cleis Press, 1999.

Magazines and information

Curve, www.curvemag.com
Diva, www.divamag.co.uk
Gay and Lesbian Medical Association, www.glma.org
Lesbians on the Loose, www.lotl.com
On our Backs, www.onourbacksmag.com
Tetu (mixed lesbian and gay magazine), www.tetu.com
365 Gay, www.365gay.com
Zero (mixed lesbian and gay magazine), www.zero-web.com

Shopping

www.aussieplayground.com.au
www.babes-n-horny.com
www.blowfish.com
www.divadirect.co.uk
www.expectations.co.uk
www.goodvibes.com
www.purplepassion.com
www.sh-womenstore.com
www.babeland.com

Picture credits

The publishers would like to thank the following sources for their kind permission to reproduce the pictures in this book.

Corbis: Bettmann: 14, 30, 37, 73, 74; /Alexander Burkatowski: 2, 21

The Bridgeman Art Library: 42, 114; /Bibliotheque Nationale, Paris, France: 12; /Christie's Images, London, UK: 6, 13; /Collection Kharbine-Tapebor, Paris, France: 62; /Galleria degli Uffizi, Florence, Italy: 68; /Gerard Nordmann, Geneva, Switzerland: 139; /Lauros/Giraudon: 22, 44; /Musée d'Orsay, Paris France: 24; /Musée du Petit Palais, Paris, France: 25, 82; / Museo Sorolla, Madrid, Spain: 112; /Museum of Fine Arts, Budapest, Hungary: 46, 49; /Private Collection: 16, 28, 56, 65, 118, 127, 141; /Pushkin Museum, Moscow, Russia: 26, 27; /Rafael Valls Gallery, London: 104; /Roy Miles Esq.: 10; /Stapleton Collection: 34, 77, 95, 108, 115, 132; /Victoria & Albert Museum, London, UK: 1, 9, 67, 90; /Wallace Collection, London, UK: 48, 55

Mary Evans Picture Library: 112

Every effort has been made to acknowledge correctly and contact the source and/or copyright holder of each picture, and Carlton Books Limited apologizes for any unintentional errors or omissions, which will be corrected in future editions of this book.